# FITNESS
## FOR THE ABSURD

Training for Geese, Groceries, and the Apocalypse.

Copyright © 2025 by Josiah Miller

All rights reserved. No part of this book may be reproduced or transmitted in any form or by any means, electronic or mechanical, including photocopying, recording, or by any information storage and retrieval system, without permission in writing from the publisher.

Published by Kokoro Health and Fitness LLC

Atlantic Beach, FL

ISBN: 979-8-90046-807-5

First Edition

Printed in the United States of America

# DEDICATION

To my hard charging 6 a.m. class.

Without you, this book wouldn't exist.

–Coach Joe

# CONTENTS

**INTRODUCTION** .................................................. iv
**HOW TO USE THIS BOOK** ........................................ viii
**DISCLAIMER** ..................................................... ix
**SECTION 1: SURVIVAL OF THE FITTEST** ................. 2
   The Mountain Goat Scramble ................................. 3
   The Angry Goose ............................................ 6
   The Shark Snack Escape ..................................... 9
   The Road Trip Log Removal ................................. 12
   The Predator Freeze ....................................... 15
   The Snake Escape Shuffle .................................. 18
**SECTION 2: EVERYDAY HEROICS** ........................... 22
   The One-Trip Wonder ....................................... 23
   The We Can't Look Like We Live Here ....................... 26
   The Stroller Sprint Save ................................... 29
   The Toddler Tackle Recovery ............................... 32
**SECTION 3: DOMESTIC TRAINING** .......................... 36
   The Baby (and Fur Baby) Retrieval .......................... 37
   The Mulch Master .......................................... 40
   The Slow Cooker Shelf Press ............................... 43
   The Couch-Crawl Plank ..................................... 46
   The DIY Furniture Store Cart Drift ......................... 49
**SECTION 4: TRAVEL & ADVENTURE** ...................... 54
   The Bucket List Stairmaster ............................... 55

The Life-in-a-Pack Trek ................................................... 58
  The Pikes Peak Warm-Up ............................................... 61
  The Concert Peek ............................................................ 64
**SECTION 5: SOCIAL SURVIVAL ................................. 68**
  The Death Grip Handshake ............................................. 69
  The Bar Lean .................................................................. 72
  The Car Seat Curl ........................................................... 75
  The Group Photo Jump ................................................... 78
  The Dance Floor Shuffle ................................................. 81
**SECTION 6: APOCALYPSE PREP ............................... 86**
  The Bunker Door Pull ..................................................... 88
  The Bridge Block Car Push ............................................ 91
  The Last Door Sledge ..................................................... 94
  The Wall Escape ............................................................. 97
  The Endurance Escape .................................................. 100
  The Apocalypse Comfort Haul ...................................... 103
**SECTION 7: NEFARIOUS ACTIVITIES ................... 108**
  The Body Drag .............................................................. 112
  The Cat Burglar ............................................................ 115
  The Buddy Haul ............................................................ 118
  The Vent Escape ........................................................... 121
**WHY FITNESS SHOULD BE FUN ............................ 124**
  Bonus Workout 1: Escape the Wreckage (Strength) ..... 128
  Bonus Workout 2: The Great Getaway (Power) ........... 131

Bonus Workout 3: The Cat Burglar (Balance & Agility) .................................................................................134

Bonus Workout 4: The Gauntlet (Endurance Circuit)....137

# THOUGHTS BEFORE YOU GO ...............................140

# Appendix A: Warm-Up, Cool-Down & Scaling ...........142

Warm-Up (5–8 Minutes) .............................................142

Cool-Down (3–5 Minutes)...........................................143

Scaling Rules (a.k.a. Don't Die Doing This) ................144

# Appendix B: The 4-Week On-Ramp..............................146

Week 1: Learn the Moves............................................147

Week 2: Add Some Spice ............................................148

Week 3: Build the Base ...............................................149

Week 4: Test the System .............................................150

Progression Rule of Thumb: ........................................151

# Appendix C: Minimal Equipment Kit............................152

The Core Kit (covers 90% of this book)........................152

The Nice-to-Have Add-Ons .........................................153

DIY / Household Substitutes........................................153

Golden Rule: ...............................................................154

# Appendix D: Glossary of Terms ....................................155

# INTRODUCTION

A few years into my career as a trainer, I started noticing something strange. On one side of the internet, you had fitness influencers screaming that if you didn't eat chicken and rice six times a day, deadlift 500 pounds, and treat your body like a part-time job, you were basically failing at life.

On the other side, you had the other 90% of the population whose lives don't revolve around the gym. People with jobs, kids, vacations, and laundry baskets overflowing like Niagara Falls. And guess what? Those people didn't have the time, or the need, to train like Olympic hopefuls just to survive a family trip to their favorite theme park.

That's when it clicked for me: fitness had gotten way too serious. The truth is, yes, being strong and capable matters. But for most people, the heaviest thing you're going to deadlift isn't a barbell loaded with four plates, it's all twelve grocery bags in one trip because there's no way you're going back to the car.

Or maybe it's your kid who, during a mid-grocery shopping meltdown, expects your gracious servitude to carry them around like royalty. That's real life, and pretending that you're not "fit" unless you're stage-ready, shredded, or an elite athlete? That's just cringe. Here's the problem: most people walk into a gym and see two things.

A bunch of machines that make you feel like cattle being herded from one pen to the next.

1. Posters or social media feeds full of fitness mutants who eat tilapia for breakfast and whose sole purpose in life seems to be flexing in better lighting.

And somewhere in the middle, the non-gym obsessed person thinks, *"Well, I guess this is fitness. I'll just sit on this machine, push this weight stack around, and hope it somehow makes me better at carrying groceries, surviving awkward family reunions, or escaping the occasional angry goose."*

Here's the catch: it won't. Because machines and bodybuilding routines aren't designed for the chaos of real life. They're designed to treat fitness like a cattle train and to make you look like someone whose only hobby is the gym, which, spoiler, you probably don't want to do.

That's where this book comes in. My goal is simple: to make you laugh, to make you think, and to secretly trick you into functional fitness. The scenarios you'll find here are absurd, sometimes ridiculous, but always rooted in reality. Could you really have to drag a body across a parking lot someday? Hopefully not. But do you need the strength and conditioning behind that movement for real life? Absolutely. And let's be honest, you're not here because you want to squat until you puke, or because you're dying to post a sweaty shirtless selfie captioned

## *"No days off"*

You're here because, deep down, you know fitness should actually mean something. Like not throwing out your back lifting a cooler full of oranges and water at your kid's soccer game. Or being able to walk up a flight of stairs without pretending to answer a "very important" phone call halfway up.

Look, I know you. You've done it. You've carried all the groceries in one trip, fingers turning purple, veins popping out of your forearms, just so you don't have to walk back to the car.

You've power-cleaned your kid off the floor in mid-tantrum. You've deadlifted a couch at least once in your life, usually at the worst possible angle, while your friend yelled, *"Pivot!"* from the other side. That's the kind of fitness this book is about. Real-life, everyday superhero strength. Except instead of spandex and saving the world, it's cargo shorts and saving your pride in front of your neighbors.

So yes, the exercises you'll find here will absolutely make you fitter, stronger, and more capable. But more importantly, they'll give you the one thing that's missing from most fitness books: the ability to laugh while you sweat.

Here's what you can expect: this book won't give you a twelve-week plan to get shredded for social media. It won't demand you sacrifice your social life in the name of macros. And it definitely won't tell you that your worth as a human being depends on your deadlift max.

What it *will* give you is something better. You'll laugh. You'll learn. You'll walk away realizing that fitness doesn't live in a weight stack or a mirror selfie — it lives in your ability to show up for your own life.

To feel confident when adventure calls. To feel capable when the unexpected happens. And maybe most importantly, to stop beating yourself up about not being "perfect" and instead start having fun while you get stronger. Because when you stop chasing someone else's idea of fitness and start building your own, even if it's through outlandish, ridiculous scenarios like outrunning an angry goose or dragging your best friend out of a bar, something amazing happens. You feel lighter. You feel stronger. You feel like, *"Yeah, I could actually handle life if it got weird."*

That's the point of this book: to give you the tools, the laughs, and the confidence to train not just for the gym… but for the beautiful, messy, unpredictable shenanigans of real life.

# HOW TO USE THIS BOOK

Congratulations, you made it past the introduction. Which means either, you're actually curious about improving your fitness, or you're just here for the goose jokes. Either way, welcome.

This book is simple: There are absurd, yet plausible scenarios. Each scenario comes with an exercise. Stick around for the bonuses at the end:

1. **A Scenario:** An absurd-but-plausible life event where you'll need this skill. (Think: "Hauling your drunk buddy out of a wedding reception before the DJ plays *Sweet Caroline* again.")

2. **The Exercise:** A straightforward breakdown of how to do it without looking like you're auditioning for a bad social media dance.

3. **Just A Tip:** Because if you can't chuckle while sweating, you're doing it wrong.

You don't have to read this book in order. Flip around. Pick the exercise that speaks to your current life crisis. Need endurance? Try the "Outrun the Goose" sprint drills. Need core strength? Head to "Couch-Crawl Plank." Need stealth? Well, there's a section for that too… but don't tell anyone.

# DISCLAIMER

This book is intended for entertainment and educational purposes only.

While the exercises and training concepts are based on legitimate fitness principles, the scenarios described, including but not limited to outrunning angry geese, escaping zombies, smuggling friends out of bars, or vaulting fences while running from the police, are fictional, exaggerated, and not to be attempted literally.

Always consult a physician or other qualified health provider before beginning any exercise program. Participation in physical activity carries inherent risks, including but not limited to injury, soreness, or embarrassment when explaining to strangers why you're practicing bear crawls in a parking lot.

The author and publisher are not liable for any injuries, mishaps, or poor life choices resulting from misuse of this material.

By reading and applying the exercises herein, you acknowledge responsibility for your own health and decisions.

To put it plainly:

- Do the exercises.
- Don't fight bears, geese, or zombies.
- Definitely don't commit crimes in the name of "training."

If you keep it playful, consistent, and safe, you'll get stronger, fitter, and maybe even laugh a little along the way. Survive. Thrive. Don't be stupid.

# SECTION 1

## SURVIVAL OF THE FITTEST

## SECTION 1: SURVIVAL OF THE FITTEST

The great outdoors. Fresh air, scenic views, and at least seven different ways to accidentally die. Nature is basically a gym that doesn't believe in waivers. Everything out there is either uphill, venomous, or plotting against your ankles.

That's why this section exists. Whether it's geese, snakes, boulders, or an entire forest deciding to block your road trip, the wilderness demands more than bicep curls and mirror selfies.

It demands sprinting when you least expect it, scrambling on all fours like a caffeinated goat, carrying things no one warned you about, and sometimes standing perfectly still while praying your deodorant holds.

The following pages will prepare you for the chaos. Will you actually be chased by a goose? Possibly. Will you wrestle a fallen log to save a vacation? Depends on your luck. But one thing's certain: train for these scenarios, and you'll walk away stronger, faster, and slightly more terrifying to anyone watching. Welcome to Wild Encounters. Try not to get bit.

## The Mountain Goat Scramble

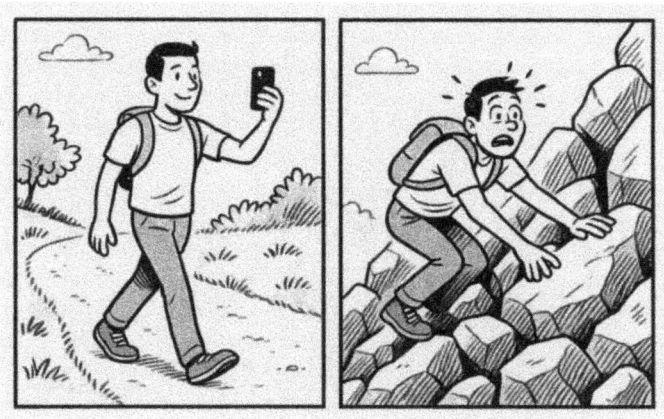

**Scenario:**
You're halfway through what was supposed to be a "casual hike" when the trail suddenly decides to become a vertical rock scramble. Two miles ago you were power-walking and taking selfies; now you're on all fours, clinging to the earth like a confused toddler who wandered onto an escalator. At this point, your best bet is to channel your inner mountain goat: low, steady, and slightly unhinged.

**The Exercise: Bear Crawl**

- Start on all fours with hands under shoulders, knees under hips.

- Hover your knees just off the ground (because mountain goats don't crawl with their shins).

- Move opposite hand and foot together; smooth and controlled, like you have great coordination.

- Keep your hips low and your core braced as you bound upward.

**Prescription:**

- 3–4 sets of 20–30 yards or until you feel like a National Geographic special.

- Rest 60–90 seconds between sets.

- Bonus round: add a light backpack for "authentic scrambling simulation."

**Form Tips:**

- Keep your back flat. You're a goat, not a scared cat.

- Small, controlled steps are better than flopping around like you're inventing new yoga poses.

- Eyes forward, not at your hands; unless you want to introduce your face to the boulder.

**Just A Tip:**

If someone films you scrambling and posts it online, just say you're "practicing primal movement." Nobody needs to know you were actually trying not to cry.

**The Angry Goose**

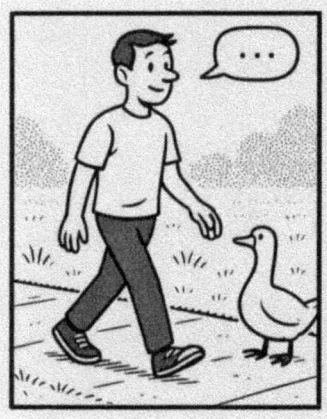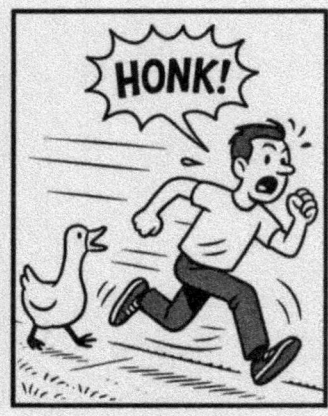

**Scenario:**
It's a beautiful day at the park. Birds are chirping, the sun is shining, and you're minding your own business… until a goose decides you're public enemy number one. Suddenly, you're not out for a peaceful walk. You're in a life-or-death footrace with a feathery velociraptor that has zero fear and an unlimited supply of rage. Your only hope? Speed.

**The Exercise: Sprint Intervals**

- Warm up with 5 minutes of light jogging or brisk walking.

- Sprint at maximum effort for 20–30 seconds (this is your "goose is on your tail" pace).

- Recover with a slow walk or light jog for 60–90 seconds.

- Repeat 6-8 rounds.

- Cool down with 5 minutes of easy walking.

**Form Tips:**

- Keep your chest up and arms pumping. The goose already has the wings, don't let it out-style you too.

- Drive your knees forward, not sideways (unless you want to look like you're doing interpretive dance mid-escape).

- Land on the balls of your feet for quick takeoff.

**Just A Tip:**
If you *actually* get chased by a goose, remember: zig-zagging doesn't work (that's alligators). Your best bet is to sprint straight, stay calm, and reflect on how interval training saved your dignity.

## The Shark Snack Escape

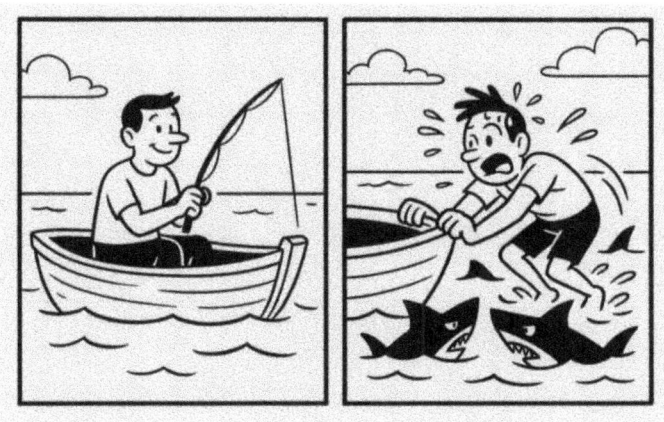

**Scenario:**

You're out on the boat, living your best life offshore, when suddenly you're not *on* the boat anymore. You're in the water. Cold. Wet. And very much surrounded by shadows that definitely don't look like friendly dolphins. At this moment, one question matters: can you haul yourself out of the water and back onto the boat, or are you about to star in the next low-budget *Shark Week* special? The pull-up decides your fate.

**The Exercise: Pull-Up**

- Find a sturdy bar (or boat rail, if you're unlucky enough to be practicing live).

- Grip it with your hands slightly wider than shoulder-width.

- Hang with arms straight and core tight, resisting the urge to thrash like bait.

- Pull your chest toward the bar by driving elbows down and back.

- Lower under control, because flopping isn't heroic.

**Prescription:**

- 4–5 sets of 3–8 reps (or as many as your shark-paranoia allows).

- Rest 2 minutes between sets, however, real rescues are not timed events.

- Bonus: Add weighted pull-ups for "great white simulation mode."

**Form Tips:**

- Don't crane your neck. Your job is to escape, not check your reflection.

- Keep your core tight. Full-body tension is your ticket out of the buffet line.

- No half reps. Sharks don't grade on effort, but people do.

**Just A Tip:**
If you can't do a pull-up, your backup plan is to outswim your slowest friend. Either way, you're training for survival.

## The Road Trip Log Removal

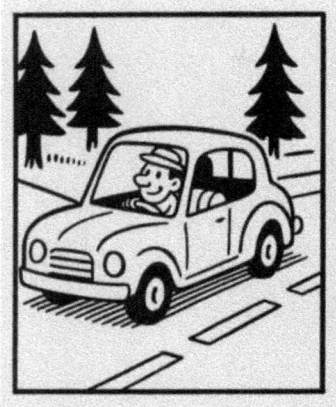 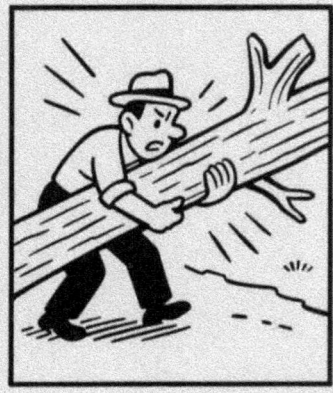

**Scenario:**
You're cruising down the highway on your epic road trip, snacks stacked, playlist on point, when the universe decides to spice things up. A giant log has crashed across the road. There's no detour, no cell service, and no chance you're explaining to everyone back home that the vacation ended because of *a tree*. The only option? Become a temporary lumberjack, lift that beast, and haul it out of the way before your snacks run out.

**The Exercise: Deadlift & Carry**

1. **Deadlift Phase:**

    - Stand with feet shoulder-width, shins close to the "log" (barbell, sandbag, or heavy object).

    - Bend at hips and knees, back flat, chest tall.

    - Grip firmly and drive through the heels to stand tall, locking it out at the top.

2. **Carry Phase:**

    - Hang onto the weight like your life depends on it, because at the very least, your toes do.

    - Walk steadily for distance (20–40 yards), keeping steps controlled.

    - Set it down safely, preferably *not* on your toes.

**Prescription:**

- 4–5 sets of: 1-3 heavy lifts + 20–40 yard carry.

- Rest 2 minutes between sets. Hauling timber isn't a race.

**Form Tips:**

- Keep the weight close. The farther away it drifts, the more likely you are to blow your discs out. (Seriously, be careful).

- Brace your core and breathe like you're trying to impress a TSA scanner.

- Small, steady steps beat "drunken penguin shuffle."

**Just A Tip:**
If anyone films you hauling a log across the road, just nod seriously and say, *"CrossFit."* No further explanation needed.

## The Predator Freeze

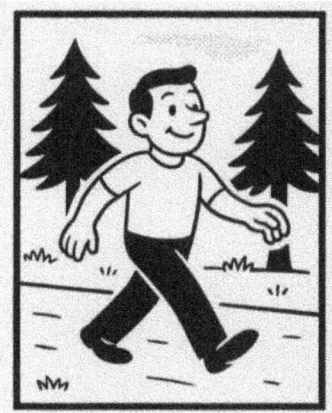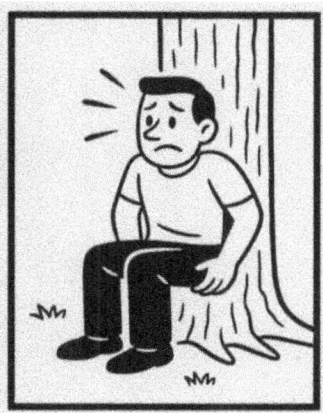

**Scenario:**
You're deep in the woods when you hear it, the snap of a twig. Your heart rate spikes, your brain flips through every nature documentary and Bigfoot conspiracy you've ever heard of, and suddenly you're convinced something is watching you. Movement? Fatal. Sound? Fatal. Your only hope is to become one with the environment: perfectly still, like a confused tourist trying to remember where they parked. Enter: the isometric hold.

**The Exercise: Wall Sit**

- Find a wall (or tree) and lean your back flat against it.

- Slide down until your thighs are parallel to the ground, knees at 90°.

- Keep your arms at your sides. No frantic waving, They can't see you if you don't move.

- Hold. And hold. And hold.

**Prescription:**

- 3–4 sets of 30–60 seconds.

- Rest 60–90 seconds between holds (or until you stop shaking like a leaf in a strong breeze).

**Form Tips:**

- Keep your knees stacked over ankles. Collapsing inwards makes you look like a folding chair.

- Brace your core. Predators can smell weakness and that burrito you had for lunch.

- Breathe slow and controlled, like you're auditioning for a meditation app.

**Just A Tip:**
If the predator doesn't leave, remember: statues never panic. Worst case, you'll just become a new trail landmark known as *"Some Dude Who Held That Wall Sit Forever."*

## The Snake Escape Shuffle

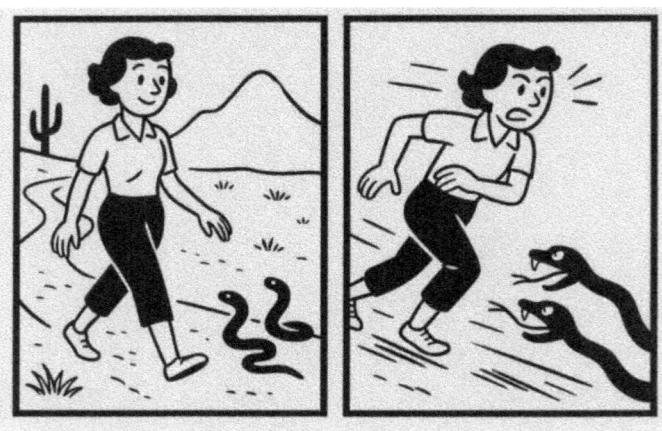

**Scenario:**
You're cruising down a sun-soaked trail when the ground suddenly slithers. Not one, not two, but an entire pit of poisonous snakes blocks your path like a living, hissing, exceptionally scary, pile of nope ropes. Running straight through? Bad idea. Turning back? Too far. Your only option: the side-to-side shuffle of someone who values their ankles and their dignity. Congratulations! You're about to discover agility you didn't know you had.

## The Exercise: Lateral Agility Shuffle

- Start in an athletic stance: feet shoulder-width apart, knees bent, weight balanced on the balls of your feet.

- Keep your chest up and core tight, like you're sneaking past a bouncer who definitely knows you're not supposed to be here.

- Push off one foot, shuffle quickly sideways, then push back the other way.

- Stay low, light, and ready to pivot like a caffeinated mongoose.

## Prescription:

- 4–5 sets of 20–30 seconds of fast shuffles.

- Rest 60 seconds between sets (snakes don't, but you should).

- Bonus: set up cones, rocks, or anything in your backyard to mimic zig-zagging past reptilian death noodles.

**Form Tips:**

- Keep your feet from crossing. Tangled legs = free lunch for the snakes.

- Stay light; the quieter you are, the less like prey you look.

- Quick bursts > long shuffles. Think "chaotic sidestep," not "interpretive dance."

**Just A Tip:**
If you trip and fall, just remember; we tried to warn you.

# SECTION 2

## EVERYDAY HEROICS

## SECTION 2: EVERYDAY HEROICS

Not all battles happen in the wild. Some of the most dangerous missions take place in your living room, driveway, or the grocery store parking lot.

Life has a way of throwing everyday chaos at you: toddlers, furniture, plastic landmines disguised as your favorite childhood building blocks; and, in those moments, your fitness is the only thing between you and disaster (or at least embarrassment and some annoying foot pain).

This section is about the unglamorous, often ridiculous situations where strength and resilience actually matter. Forget perfect lighting and protein shakes.

This is about surviving your child's construction project without losing your balance, carrying all the groceries in one hand while your toddler demands to be carried in the other, and launching yourself off the ground mid-burpee to save a runaway stroller.

Will you ever need to perform a flawless Turkish Get-Up while holding a child overhead? Maybe not. But if you can, you'll be ready for just about anything domestic life throws at you and you'll look like a superhero in the process.

Everyday life is messy. Everyday life is unpredictable. And sometimes, everyday life is the hardest workout you'll ever do.

**The One-Trip Wonder**

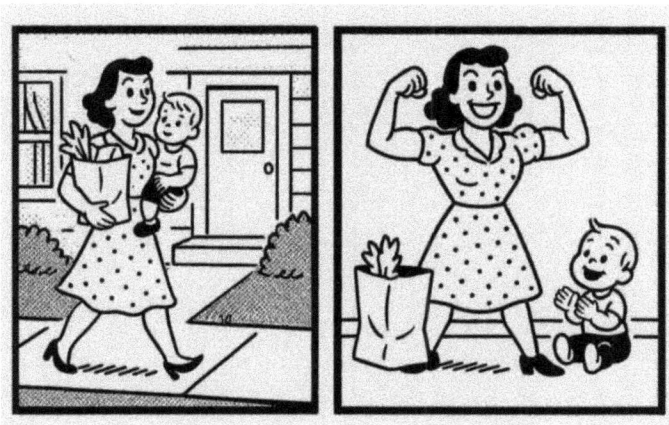

**Scenario:**
It's the end of a long day. You've got 47 pounds of groceries in one hand, a squirming toddler clamped to the other, and a front door that suddenly feels like the Fort Knox of doorknobs. You refuse to make two trips, because two trips means weakness, so you grit your teeth and suitcase-carry your way to household glory.

The only thing between you and victory (and melting ice cream) is your grip strength, core stability, and the ability to unlock a door with one functioning hand.

**The Exercise: Suitcase Carry**

- Grab one heavy weight in one hand (dumbbell, kettlebell, suitcase, or bag of shamefully large frozen pizzas).

- Stand tall, shoulders level. Don't lean like the Leaning Tower of Pisa.

- Walk forward in a straight line while resisting the urge to tilt sideways.

- Switch hands each set unless you actually enjoy chronic back pain.

**Prescription:**

- 3–4 sets of 30–40 yards per hand.

- Rest 60–90 seconds between carries.

- Bonus: Carry your child at the same time to perform the coveted "SIT-C Method" (Simultaneous Infant Transport and Carry)

**Form Tips:**

- Keep your chest up. Confidence counts when neighbors are watching.

- Brace your core like you're about to sneeze in a library.

- Walk steady; wobbling makes you look like a drunk pirate.

**Just A Tip:**
If you drop the groceries while unlocking the door, just yell "hot potato!" and pretend it was part of your plan so people think you're fun. If performing the SIT-C Method, good parenting is dropping the groceries….right?

## The We Can't Look Like We Live Here

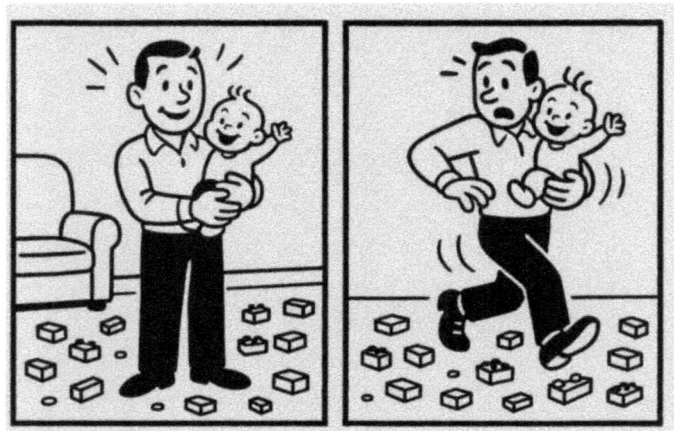

**Scenario:**
The living room looks like a toy factory exploded. Tiny, colorful, sharp, evil little bricks whose mission is creating joy and foot-destroying pain, are scattered across the floor like a minefield. To make matters worse, your child insists on being carried like royalty while you clean up their plastic empire. Now you're stuck doing deep lunges, one hand scooping up demonic little squares, the other hand balancing a toddler who's offering zero help and maximum commentary. This isn't a workout, it's parental survival.

## The Exercise: Forward Lunge

- Stand tall with a child (or heavy object) balanced on one hip.

- Step one leg forward, lowering until your front knee is at 90° and your back knee hovers above the ground.

- Keep your chest tall and your construction hand free.

- Push off your front foot to return to standing.

- Repeat, alternating legs and watch out for stray bricks.

## Prescription:

- 3–4 sets of 8–10 lunges per leg.

- Rest 60–90 seconds between sets (or until your hip regains feeling).

- Bonus: Scatter actual objects (not little bricks, you deserve better) to "collect" while you lunge. Or, just clean your floor… because you live there.

**Form Tips:**

- Keep your core braced. Nothing says bad parenting like toppling a child mid-lunge.

- Knee over toes will not kill you, but focus on hitting good form with every single rep, it matters.

- Don't rush; wobbling here means face-planting into the toy box.

**Just A Tip:**
If you step on a tiny brick from hell, just scream dramatically, your neighbors will assume you're either being mugged or doing extreme HIIT. Both are accurate.

## The Stroller Sprint Save

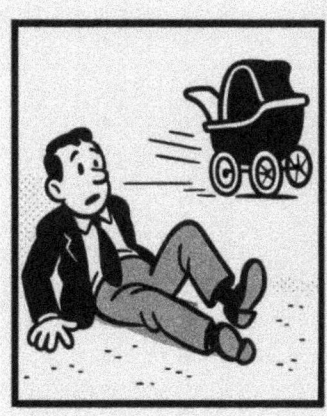 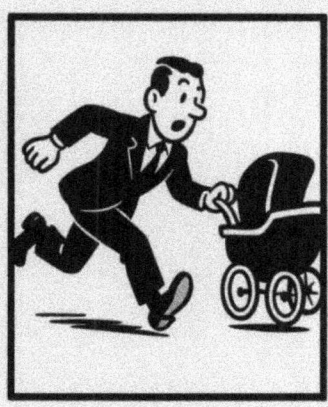

**Scenario:**
It's a picture-perfect day. You're strolling peacefully with the baby when fate decides to spice things up. Your toe catches the one crack in the sidewalk, and down you go. As you hit the ground, you see it– the stroller rolling away, wheels locked on course for the busiest intersection in town. There's no time to think, only one option: hit the ground, pop up like your life depends on it, and sprint into action. In other words... the burpee just became the most important exercise of your parenting career.

**The Exercise: Burpee**

- Start standing tall, like a responsible adult.

- Drop into a squat and kick your legs back into a plank.

- Lower your chest to the ground (bonus points if you scream internally).

- Explosively push yourself back up, jump your feet forward, and launch into the air.

- Land ready to sprint, because the stroller won't wait for your cooldown.

**Prescription:**

- 3–4 sets of 8–12 reps.

- Rest 90 seconds between sets. You're going to need it because this one burns like daycare tuition.

- Bonus: Add a 20-yard sprint after each burpee to practice the "try not to be a bad parent baby-chasing combo."

**Form Tips:**

- Keep your core braced, don't flop like a fish out of water.

- Land soft on the jump. You're saving a baby, not auditioning for *Riverdance*.

- Pace yourself; the stroller might roll far, but you don't want to gas out mid-rescue.

**Just A Tip:**
If bystanders stare, just shout *"functional parenting!"* mid-burpee and keep going.

## The Toddler Tackle Recovery

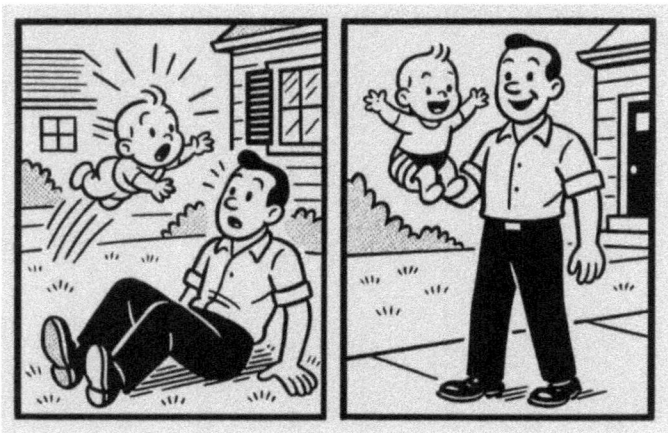

**Scenario:**

It's a peaceful evening at home. You're on the floor, maybe stretching, maybe just existing. Suddenly, out of nowhere, a 30-pound toddler launches themselves at you like a caffeinated linebacker.

Suddenly, you're pinned. You're dazed. You're questioning your life choices. The only way back to dignity? Rising from the floor like a phoenix from the ashes, with grace, balance, and strength; all while holding your squirming opponent overhead like a baby lion in Africa.

## The Exercise: Turkish Get-Up

1. Lie on your back, one arm holding a weight (or child) straight up toward the ceiling.

2. Bend the same-side knee, keeping the foot flat on the ground.

3. Roll up onto your opposite elbow, then hand, keeping your "precious cargo" balanced overhead.

4. Sweep your leg under into a kneeling position.

5. Stand up tall like the conquering hero you are.

6. Reverse each step to return to the floor. Bonus points for not dropping the kid or the kettlebell.

## Prescription:

- 3–5 sets of 3–5 reps per side.

- Rest 90–120 seconds between sets. The stakes are high and this is not a race.

- Bonus: Try it with a backpack full of random household junk for "real-life simulation mode."

**Form Tips:**

- Eyes on the weight overhead, because nothing says "bad day" like a kettlebell to the forehead.

- Move slow and controlled. Speed is for goose sprints, not toddler tackles.

- Keep your core tight. Flopping = toddler victory.

**Just A Tip:**
If you can stand up from the floor holding a wriggling toddler overhead, congratulations, you're now officially stronger than half the parents at the playground.

PS: Watch out for ceiling fans... don't ask.

# SECTION 3

## DOMESTIC TRAINING

## SECTION 3: DOMESTIC TRAINING

Forget the wilderness or world travel, the most dangerous terrain you'll ever face is your own home. Domestic life is an obstacle course disguised as "chores." One minute you're rescuing a child who's decided the floor is lava, the next you're wheelbarrowing mulch like an unpaid landscaper, and before you know it, you're locked in mortal combat with a slow cooker that somehow weighs more than your dog.

And let's not forget our favorite DIY furniture store, the final boss of domestic chaos. Sure, you survived the maze of fake apartments, but the real test comes in the parking lot.

Four-wheel steering carts that drift like rally cars, loaded with flat-pack furniture and questionable life choices, will teach you more about core stability than any ab machine ever invented.

This section is about training for survival in the wildest place of all: your home (and everything you drag back into it). Squats, deadlifts, presses, planks, even cart drifts.

These aren't just exercises, they're the difference between looking like you've got it together and admitting defeat to a pile of mulch or a runaway labrador.

Domestic life will test you. This section will prepare you. Just don't expect it to make furniture assembly any easier.

## The Baby (and Fur Baby) Retrieval

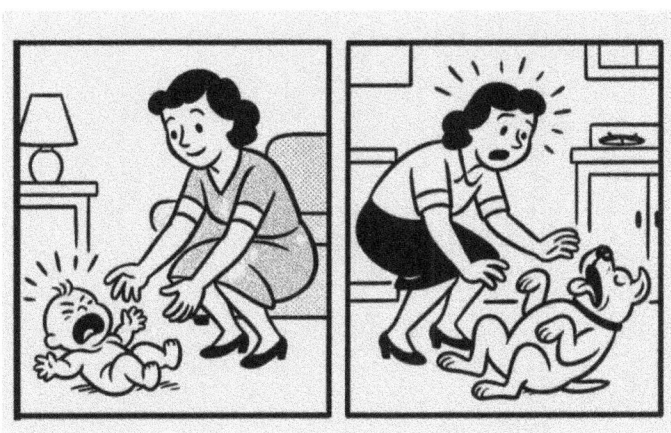

**Scenario:**
You're just trying to enjoy five minutes of peace when disaster strikes: your child decides gravity is optional and launches themselves onto the floor, or your dog collapses dramatically in the middle of the kitchen like it's auditioning for an Oscar.

Neither of them plans to get up on their own. And since society frowns on leaving them there until they figure it out, your only option is to squat down and pick them up like the functional adult you pretend to be.

**The Exercise: Bodyweight (or Weighted) Squat**

- Stand with your feet shoulder-width apart, toes slightly out like you're ready for action.

- Sit your hips back and bend your knees, lowering until your thighs are parallel to the ground.

- Keep your chest tall and your heels planted, no toddler faceplants or dog drops allowed.

- Push through your heels to stand tall, ideally while scooping up the child or fur child in one smooth motion.

**Prescription:**

- 3–4 sets of 10–15 reps.

- Rest 60 seconds between sets (or until the dog decides to "help").

- Bonus: Add a weight (kettlebell, child, or small-to-medium dog) for realism.

**Form Tips:**

- Knees track over toes, not inwards, unless you want to invent a new dance move.

- Keep your core tight like you're bracing to watch your toddler throw food at the wall.

- Depth matters: no "half squats." Kids and dogs don't levitate halfway up.

**Just A Tip:**
If you misjudge and groan loudly mid-squat, just tell everyone it's "power breathing." Nobody needs to know your spine is negotiating with your incredibly tight hips.

**The Mulch Master**

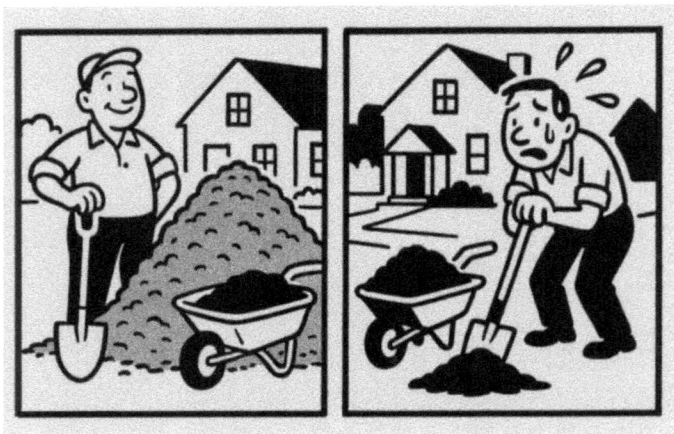

**Scenario:**
It's Saturday morning, which means one thing: your spouse has a new "totally easy project" planned. Today's task? Wheelbarrow several metric tons of mulch across the yard for the garden that apparently can't survive without it.

You agree because of love, but two trips in you realize this is less gardening and more unpaid labor. Your hamstrings, glutes, and lower back are the only things standing between you and becoming mulch yourself. Time for the Romanian Deadlift.

**The Exercise: Romanian Deadlift (RDL)**

- Stand tall with feet hip-width apart, weight (barbell, dumbbells, or "imaginary wheelbarrow handles") in front of you.

- With a soft bend in the knees, hinge at the hips and lower the weight down your thighs, keeping your back flat and chest proud.

- Lower until you feel your hamstrings stretch tighter than your weekend schedule.

- Drive your hips forward to stand tall, finishing strong enough to keep your marriage intact.

**Prescription:**

- 3–4 sets of 8–10 reps.

- Rest 90 seconds between sets, or long enough to pretend you're "hydrating" and definitely not stalling.

- Bonus: Do this with your wheelbarrow to simulate the "real life" version.

**Form Tips:**

- Back straight. Rounding turns this into chiropractic cosplay.

- Keep the weight close, the farther it drifts, the more likely your spine will file a complaint.

- Move slow and controlled; flopping forward makes you look like the mulch already won.

**Just A Tip:**
If your spouse questions why it's taking you so long, just say you're "building functional strength which requires adequate rest periods." They'll still hand you another wheelbarrow load, but at least you'll sound like a pro.

## The Slow Cooker Shelf Press

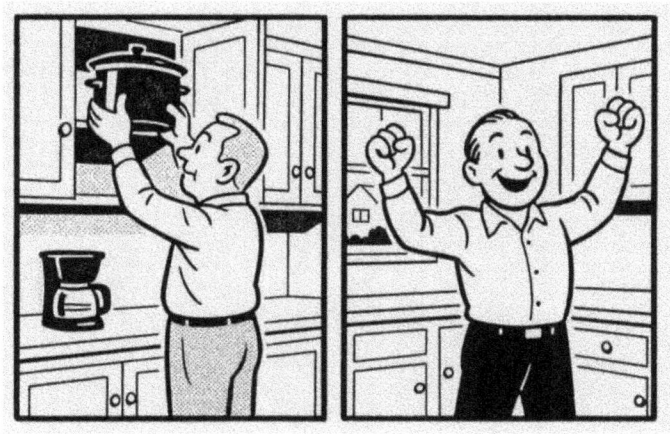

**Scenario:**
Your kitchen cabinets are already packed tighter than a holiday buffet when your spouse casually says, *"Just put the slow cooker on the top shelf."* The problem? This "slow cooker" weighs roughly the same as a small car engine and is shaped like it was designed by someone who hates ergonomics.

There's no easy angle, no safe grip, and no option to say no, because apparently chili night depends on your shoulders of steel. Time for the overhead press.

**The Exercise: Overhead Press**

- Stand with feet shoulder-width apart, weight (barbell, dumbbells, or small appliance) at shoulder height.

- Brace your core like you're holding a giant bowl of hot cheese soup over your head.

- Press the weight straight overhead until your arms are fully extended.

- Lower with control. Smashing the slow cooker into the counter is not an acceptable finish.

**Prescription:**

- 3–4 sets of 8–12 reps.

- Rest 90 seconds between sets. Heavy cookware isn't forgiving.

- Bonus: Use awkward household items (boxes, laundry baskets, or yes, your actual slow cooker) for "realism training."

**Form Tips:**

- Don't arch your back; this is strength training, not the limbo.

- Keep wrists straight; bending them turns the press into wrist roulette.

- Move in a vertical line, not forward; unless you *want* to explain why there's a slow cooker-sized hole in the drywall.

**Just A Tip:**
If you get it up there safely, pause, flex, and say, *"Dinner is served."* Congratulations, you just PR'd in domestic survival.

## The Couch-Crawl Plank

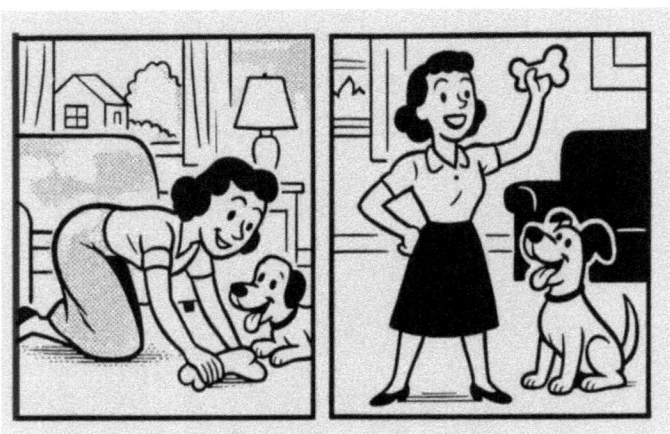

**Scenario:**
Your dog has once again launched its favorite toy into the one place it knows you can't reach: under the couch. You try the broom trick and manage to knock it all over the place, wishing this stick had hands.

That leaves just one option: drop down, stretch as far as humanly possible, and hold a plank while you fish around like a mechanic working under a car looking for the fabled 10mm socket. Welcome to the ultimate test of core strength and patience.

**The Exercise: Plank**

- Start face down on the floor, elbows under shoulders, forearms flat.
- Lift your body so only forearms and toes touch the ground.
- Keep your body in a straight line from head to heels, no sagging, no piking (butt up in the air).
- Hold while reaching forward with one arm like a human claw machine.

**Prescription:**

- 3–4 sets of 30–60 second holds.
- Rest 60–90 seconds between attempts, or long enough to yell at the dog for moral support.
- Bonus: Add toy retrieval reps mid-hold for "real-life authenticity."

**Form Tips:**

- Keep hips level, if they drop, so does your pride.

- Brace your core like you're trying to keep laughter in at a board meeting.

- Eyes down, not wandering; otherwise you'll lose track of the toy. Then you are no better than the broom handle.

**Just A Tip:**
If you finally retrieve the toy only for your dog to immediately shove it back under. You will be fine, the world record plank is over 8 hours… you've got this!

## The DIY Furniture Store Cart Drift

**Scenario:**
You went to everyone's favorite Swedish furniture store to "get some decoration inspiration." Two hours later, you're wheeling a cart piled higher than a shopper on Black Friday in 2008, stacked with boxes that look like Tetris on hard mode.

That's when you remember: These carts have four-wheel steering from hell, because making you build your own furniture wasn't a big enough clue on how they feel about you. Suddenly you're not pushing a cart, you're piloting a runaway go-kart down a hilly parking lot, narrowly avoiding bystanders, parked cars, and your own obituary. The only thing keeping you from disaster? Core strength and steering control worthy of a Tokyo drift car driver.

**The Exercise: Standing Core Twist**

- Stand with feet shoulder-width apart, holding a weight (medicine ball, dumbbell, or small flat-pack box) at chest height.

- Engage your core, rotate your torso to one side like you're wrenching your cart back from certain doom.

- Return to center, then rotate to the opposite side. Go fast and squeeze your abs hard to stop before rotating back.

- Keep hips facing forward; all the power comes from your core, not flailing arms.

**Prescription:**

- 3–4 sets of 12–15 twists per side.

- Rest 60 seconds between sets (long enough to swear off flat-pack furniture forever).

- Bonus: Try it while holding something awkward and lopsided, like a lamp named *Sven*.

**Form Tips:**

- Don't let your knees drift, this isn't salsa class, it's preparation.

- Keep your core tight, loose abs lead to a 68% increase in cart crash risk.

- Control the range. Dramatic over-rotations belong in action movies, not parking lots.

**Just A Tip:**
If you drift wildly out of control and nearly take out a parked car, make some race car sounds and let your inner child free.

# SECTION 4

## TRAVEL & ADVENTURE

# SECTION 4: TRAVEL & ADVENTURE

Vacations are supposed to be relaxing, but in reality, they're just fitness tests without enough snacks. Every trip promises "unforgettable memories" but usually delivers burning legs, heavy packs, and at least one moment where you consider calling for a rescue helicopter.

This section is your training guide for the chaos of adventure. Think of it as a survival manual for bucket-list trips that don't care about your comfort zone. You'll climb endless stone steps carved into the Grand Canyon like Mother Nature's personal StairMaster.

You'll strap on a pack loaded with more regrets than water and discover the suffering known as rucking. You'll reach the summit of Pikes Peak in shorts and a t-shirt, only to realize summer doesn't exist up there and your best bet is flailing through jumping jacks to stay warm.

And when you finally unwind at a concert, you'll discover the tallest people on earth have gathered in front of you, forcing you into calf raises just to catch a glimpse of the stage.

Adventure isn't about Instagram-worthy photos. It's about surviving the climb, the weight, the cold, and the crowds. Do these exercises, and your reward won't just be strength and stamina. It'll be the ability to say, *"Yeah, I made it,"* without needing to explain how close you came to being airlifted out.

## The Bucket List Stairmaster

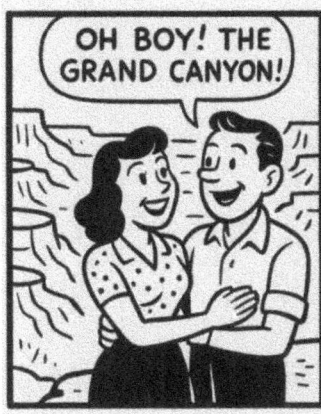 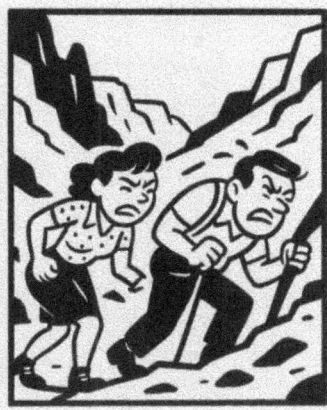

**Scenario:**
You've finally made it to your bucket-list hike: the Grand Canyon, South Rim to Bright Angel Trail, staring down miles of unforgiving switchbacks and rocky stair-steps that climb out of the canyon like stone serpents.

What the guidebooks don't highlight? The part where hikers get airlifted out for "medical emergencies" multiple times a day, because your quads forgot they'd signed up for this. Now, every step up feels like negotiating peace treaties with gravity. This isn't just a hike; it's a vertical showdown.

**The Exercise: Step-Up**

- Find a sturdy surface, like a shin-busting step or a boulder carrying "Grand Canyon" vibes.

- Place your foot firmly on the surface, press through the heel, drive your body upward.

- Stand tall at the top for a split second, surveying your future suffering (or the view, whichever motivates you more).

- Step down under control.

- Alternate legs each rep unless you want one leg to feel like it's on strike.

**Prescription:**

- 3–4 sets of 10–12 reps per leg (or until you're considering launching an emergency flare).

- Rest 60–90 seconds between sets; like your quads, your lungs need a breather too.

- Bonus: Strap on a pack to simulate hauling all your regrets (and water) up those canyon steps.

**Form Tips:**

- Whole foot on the step. Dangling toes equal slow-motion faceplants.

- Don't push off with the back leg. It's not a hopscotch contest, it's pure uphill grind.

- Keep your chest up, hunching just puts you at risk of becoming a footnote in someone else's rescue story.

**Just A Tip:**
If you start fantasizing about that rescue helicopter, remember: getting airlifted out of the Grand Canyon costs more than your entire vacation. It's best to be prepared and work those step-ups.

## The Life-in-a-Pack Trek

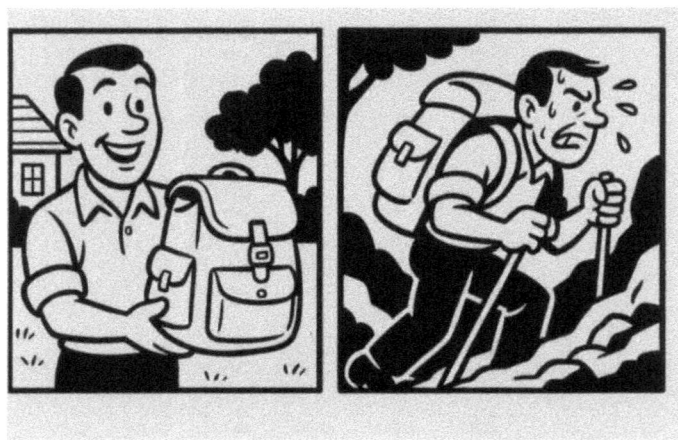

**Scenario:**
Nothing says "adventure" like strapping your entire existence onto your back and calling it fun. Hiking boots laced, pack loaded with 30 pounds of snacks, extra socks, and that one "just in case" item you'll never use, you set off down the trail.

Five miles later, you realize rucking is basically paying money to suffer slowly under a backpack that whispers, *"You should've bought the cumberbund."*

**The Exercise: Rucking (Weighted Hike/Walk)**

- Load a backpack with weight (start light: water jugs, books, or canned beans you'll never eat).

- Strap it snug to your back, sloppy packs mean sloppy posture.

- Walk briskly for distance or time, keeping your stride smooth and controlled.

- Bonus points if you mutter survival movie quotes along the way.

**Prescription:**

- 1–2 sessions per week, 20–45 minutes.

- Start with 10–20% of your bodyweight; build up slowly unless you like chiropractor visits.

- Bonus: Train on hills or stairs to simulate "Grand Canyon Lite."

**Form Tips:**

- Keep your core braced and shoulders back. Don't morph into the Hunchback of Trail-dom.

- Swing your arms naturally, over-striding just makes you look like an Olympic power walker.

- Break it in slowly. Rucking is not a sprint, it's an endurance negotiation with discomfort.

**Just A Tip:**
If you can still feel your shoulders after mile five, GOOD, you are ready to go up in weight. If you can't, welcome to the club.

Membership benefits include sweaty shirts, sore traps, and enough calories burnt for that churro you have been craving all day.

## The Pikes Peak Warm-Up

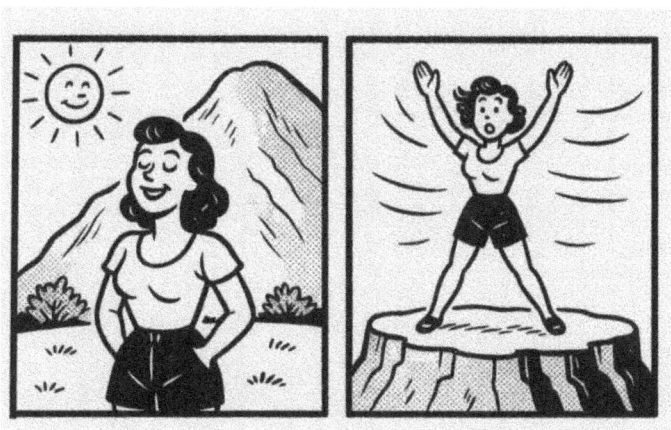

**Scenario:**
It seemed like a good idea at the trailhead: sunny skies, warm breeze, summer vibes. "We're totally ready for this," you said, brimming with confidence and loads of granola bars. Fast forward a few thousand feet, and welcome to the top of Pikes Peak, where summer is dead, winter is alive, and your body suddenly realizes how woefully under-prepared you are. Before you freeze solid and get mistaken for modern art, your only option is to warm up fast with the timeless exercise, jumping jacks.

## The Exercise: Jumping Jack

- Stand tall, feet together, arms at your sides.

- Jump your feet out wide as you swing your arms overhead.

- Jump feet back together as your arms return to your sides.

- Repeat rhythmically until your lungs file a complaint.

## Prescription:

- 3–4 sets of 30–60 seconds.

- Rest 30 seconds between sets (not that the altitude will let you).

- Bonus: Try it with a pack still on, nothing says "prepared" like slapping yourself in the face with your own straps.

**Form Tips:**

- Land soft. Stomping at 14,000 feet just makes you sound like an angry elk.

- Keep your arms moving in sync. Flailing turns this into an interpretive dance.

- Control your breathing, or at least try, while the thin air laughs at you.

**Just A Tip:**
If a tourist side-eyes you for doing jumping jacks on the summit, just make unusually long eye contact until the problem goes away.

## The Concert Peek

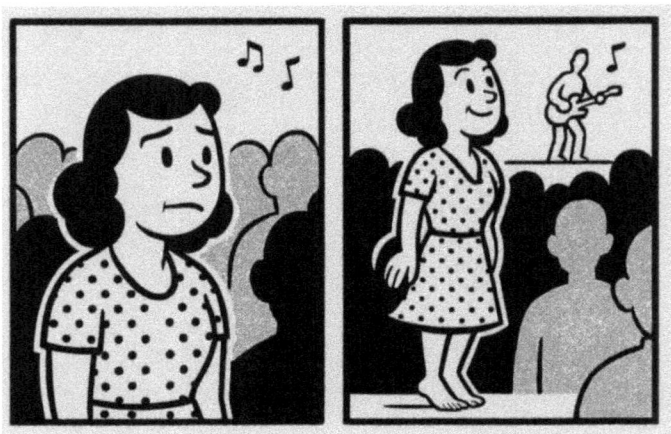

**Scenario:**
You're finally at the concert of your dreams. The lights flash, the music hits, and the crowd goes wild. There's only one problem: you're stuck behind a human redwood forest.

No matter how you angle it, all you see are shoulders, ponytails, and the back of someone's sweaty neck. Your only chance to glimpse the stage before the encore is to channel your inner mountain goat, springing up on your toes again and again until your calves catch fire and you see salvation or at least the lead singer's hairline.

## The Exercise: Standing Calf Raise

- Stand tall, feet hip-width apart.

- Press through the balls of your feet, lifting your heels as high as you can like you're clawing for oxygen at altitude.

- Hold for a second at the top and drink in that half-second view of the band.

- Lower slowly, because collapsing like a fainting goat is not the vibe.

## Prescription:

- 3–5 sets of 15–20 reps.

- Rest 45–60 seconds between sets (time it with the drummer's solo).

- Bonus: Try single-leg raises for an advanced "ballerina mode."

**Form Tips:**

- Don't bounce. Pogo-stick impressions won't help you here.

- Keep your movements smooth and steady; jerky jumps just make you a hazard.

- Squeeze your calves at the top like the fate of your ticket price depends on it, because it does.

**Just A Tip:**
If your view is still blocked, just accept reality: you could always ask someone to get on their shoulders which will require core strength - see the DIY Furniture Store Scenario.

# SECTION 5

SOCIAL SURVIVAL

## SECTION 5: SOCIAL SURVIVAL

Gyms won't tell you this, but some of the hardest workouts you'll ever face happen at weddings, reunions, and backyard barbecues. Social events are basically obstacle courses with bad music and higher stakes. One weak handshake, one failed jump in a group photo, one collapse at the bar and you'll never live it down in the group chat.

This section is your playbook for staying strong in the chaos of human interaction. Grip training so your handshake doesn't feel like a limp noodle. Core stability so you can lean casually at the bar without toppling over like a poorly constructed tower of cards.

Biceps strong enough to haul a car seat or hold someone's bag without your arm shaking like a leaf in the wind. Jump squats so you actually get airtime in that photo instead of looking like you tripped. And agility drills so you can dodge elbows and escape the dance floor before someone demands the Macarena.

You may never wrestle a bear or sprint from geese, but you *will* face these moments. And when you do, your training will save you from humiliation. Welcome to Social Survival, proof that fitness isn't just about muscles. It's about not becoming a family meme.

## The Death Grip Handshake

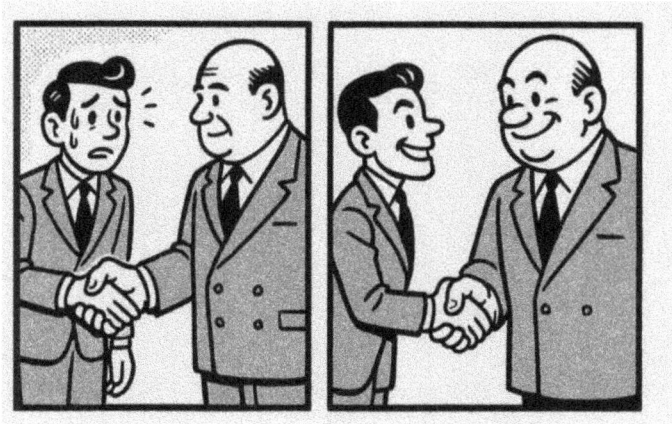

**Scenario:**

You're meeting your partner's dad for the first time. He extends his hand, it's massive, calloused, and already radiating dominance. This is no ordinary handshake; this is a duel. If your grip is weak, you'll forever be remembered as *"the limp noodle."*

If your grip is strong, you earn respect, or at least the right to date in peace. The only thing between you and future family holidays is the crushing power of your forearms.

## The Exercise: Farmer's Hold (Grip Strength)

- Grab two heavy dumbbells, kettlebells, or grocery bags full of way too many snacks.

- Stand tall, arms at your sides, shoulders back.

- Hold until your grip fails or your soul leaves your body.

- Repeat. Because awkward holiday dinners are forever.

## Prescription:

- 3–4 sets of 30–60 second holds.

- Rest 60–90 seconds between sets while practicing small talk.

- Bonus: Try single-hand holds for the "in-law challenge."

**Form Tips:**

- Don't hunch forward. Nothing says "beta" like rounded shoulders.

- Breathe steady, shallow gasps look suspicious.

- Squeeze hard. Pretend you're trying to crush your mortal enemy's dreams.

**Just A Tip:**

If you lose the handshake battle, just nod and say, *"Nice grip, sport."* This will assert your dominance and definitely not backfire.

PS. If you haven't already, read the disclaimer.

## The Bar Lean

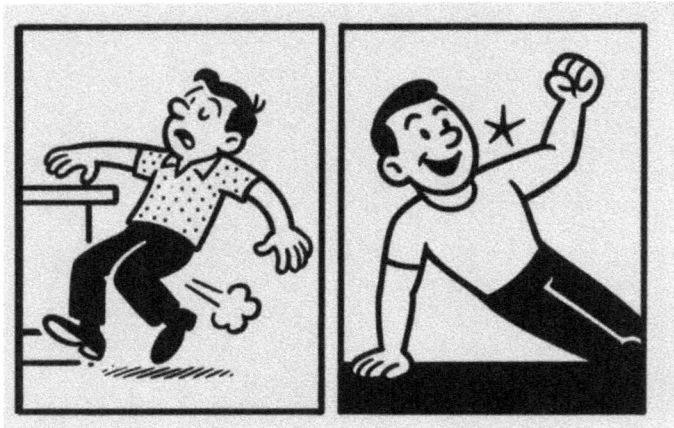

**Scenario:**
You're at the bar trying to look cool, casual, and collected. You lean against the counter like you own the place, except your core is weaker than your drink order.

Suddenly, instead of James Bond, you're collapsing like a folding lawn chair. Your only salvation? The side plank: the difference between "effortlessly chill" and "that guy who fell off the bar stool without even drinking."

**The Exercise: Side Plank**

- Lie on your side, elbow directly under your shoulder, legs stacked.

- Lift your hips until your body forms a straight line from head to heels.

- Hold, bracing your core like paparazzi just spotted you.

- Switch sides unless you want a six-pack on one side and a dad bod on the other.

**Prescription:**

- 3–4 sets of 20–45 seconds per side.

- Rest 60 seconds between sets, or time it with a bartender ignoring you.

- Bonus: Add hip dips for advanced "bar swagger training."

**Form Tips:**

- Keep your hips high, because those hips don't lie.

- Don't let your shoulder collapse; this isn't a chiropractic experiment.

- Eyes forward, not down, because casual confidence doesn't involve staring at the floor.

**Just A Tip:**
If you wobble mid-lean, just smirk and say, *"I'm on tonight...you know my hips don't lie...."* Works every time.

## The Car Seat Curl

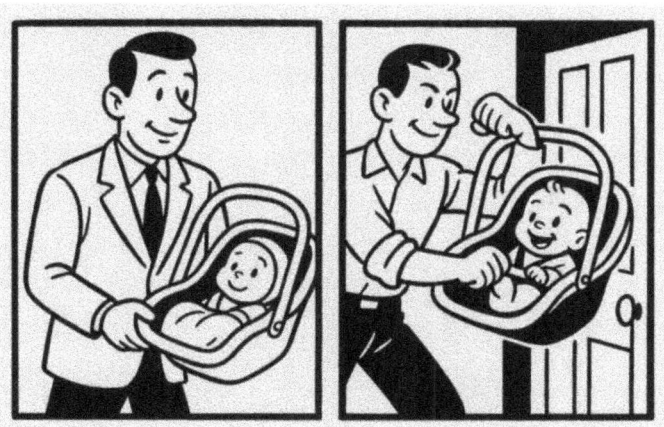

**Scenario:**
Few things test the human spirit like lugging a child strapped into a car seat. It's shaped like a medieval torture device, awkwardly balanced, and always heavier than you remember.

Add in the fact that you're hauling it with one arm while trying to unlock the front door with the other, and suddenly your biceps are the only thing keeping you from dropping both your kid and your dignity.

**The Exercise: Bicep Curl**

- Stand tall with a weight in one hand (dumbbell, suitcase, or, yes, a car seat if you're feeling brave).

- Keep your elbow glued to your side.

- Curl the weight up toward your shoulder in one smooth motion.

- Lower slowly; no parent has ever "thrown" a car seat gracefully.

**Prescription:**

- 3–4 sets of 8–12 reps per arm.

- Rest 60–90 seconds between sets (or however long it takes your toddler to stop asking "why").

- Bonus: Try a few curls while holding something in your other hand to mimic true "parent struggle mode."

**Form Tips:**

- Keep your reps smooth, nobody wants shaken baby syndrome.

- Don't shrug your shoulders, you're not reenacting *The Hunchback of Notre Dame.*

- Control the weight; jerking it up only guarantees toy shrapnel flying out of the seat.

**Just A Tip:**

If anyone questions why you're curling a car seat, just smile and say, *"Parenting is my workout plan."* They'll believe you.

## The Group Photo Jump

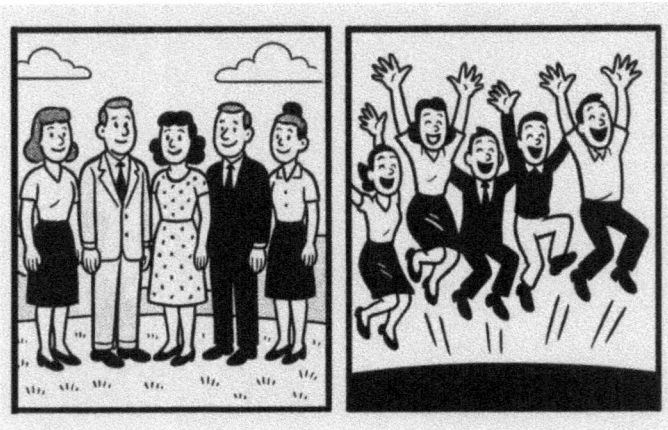

**Scenario:**
You're at a wedding, family reunion, or work event when someone yells, *"Okay, everybody jump on three!"* Suddenly you're not just in a photo, you're in a competition.

If your vertical is weak, you'll be the sad blur two inches off the ground while everyone else looks like basketball all-stars. The only way to avoid eternal group chat shame is to train your jump squats until you can levitate like you mean it.

**The Exercise: Jump Squat**

- Start standing with feet shoulder-width apart.

- Drop into a squat, loading your legs like coiled springs.

- Explode upward, launching yourself into the air like your reputation depends on it.

- Land softly, bend your knees, and reset for the next rep.

**Prescription:**

- 3–4 sets of 8–12 reps.

- Rest 90 seconds between sets (or until your legs forgive you).

- Bonus: Practice shouting "Wooooo!" mid-air for true photo realism.

**Form Tips:**

- Keep your chest up. You're going for "majestic," not "face-first nosedive."

- Use your arms for lift; floppy arms equal floppy jump.

- Land soft; stomping looks less like fun and more like a toddler tantrum.

**Just A Tip:**
If you still barely get off the ground, just own it, crouch dramatically and tell everyone you were "going for artistic depth."

## The Dance Floor Shuffle

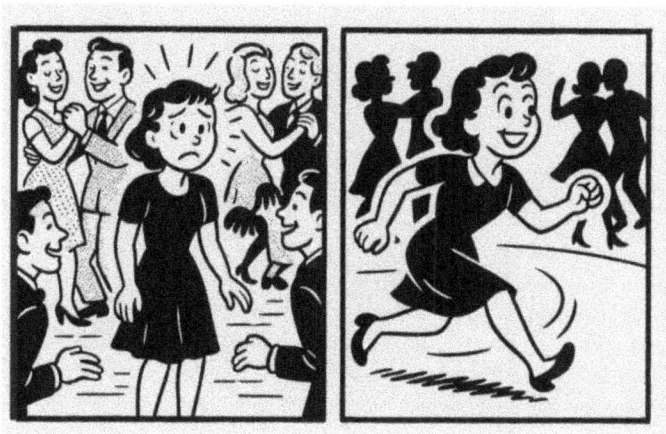

**Scenario:**

The DJ drops a banger, the dance floor fills up, and suddenly you're in the middle of it, trapped between an enthusiastic aunt doing the Macarena and a friend who thinks "flailing wildly" counts as rhythm.

Your only hope of survival is to shuffle, dodge, and weave your way through the human stampede without spilling your drink or catching an elbow to the teeth. This isn't dancing, this is agility training at its finest.

**The Exercise: Lateral Agility Shuffle**

- Start in an athletic stance: knees bent, feet shoulder-width apart, weight on the balls of your feet.

- Push off one foot and shuffle sideways like you're dodging a sweaty uncle's interpretive spin.

- Switch directions quickly, staying light and controlled.

- Keep your chest up, your dignity's already at risk, don't add a faceplant to your core memories.

**Prescription:**

- 4–5 sets of 20–30 seconds.

- Rest 60 seconds between sets, or use the time to grab another drink.

- Bonus: Add cones, chairs, or people with questionable moves as obstacles to dodge.

**Form Tips:**

- Stay low. The lower you are, the faster you can slide out of disaster.

- Don't cross your feet. Tripping here is how legends (of shame) are made.

- Quick bursts beat long slides; think "smooth sidestep," not "ice skater meltdown."

**Just A Tip:**
If anyone asks what you're doing, just shrug mid-shuffle and say, *"Dance defense."* Instant respect.

# SECTION 6

## APOCALYPSE PREP

# SECTION 6: APOCALYPSE PREP

Sure, gyms are nice. But when the world ends, there won't be dumbbells, treadmills, or protein shakes, there will be chaos.

And the only thing standing between you and becoming zombie chow is whether or not you trained for the *real* big lifts: pulling doors shut, shoving cars off bridges, smashing through barricades, climbing walls, running for your life, and carrying the one item you refuse to leave behind (probably snacks).

This section is about survival fitness in its purest form. Rows become the strength to slam bunker doors. Sled pushes mean the difference between crossing the bridge or taking a swim in a hypothermia river.

Sledgehammer slams teach you how to break through barricades before the horde breaks through you. Pull-ups and rope climbs? That's your ticket up and over the wall when the street is swarming.

Zone 2 cardio keeps your heart efficient enough to actually outlast the chase. And the weighted front carry? Well… sometimes survival means hugging your apocalypse comfort item and hauling it to safety, because no one's facing the end of the world without snacks.

Will you ever need this exact training? Hopefully not. But if the big one hits, you'll be ready. And even if it doesn't, you'll be stronger, tougher, and just a little scarier to anyone watching you slam a sledgehammer into a tire like it owes you money.

Welcome to Apocalypse Prep. Survive the chaos, save the snacks.

## The Bunker Door Pull

**Scenario:**

It finally happened. Zombies, aliens, or maybe just your HOA coming for blood. Either way, you've made it to the bunker. One problem: the door weighs about 600 pounds, it's stuck halfway shut, and your survival depends on ripping it closed before anything squeezes through.

This is no cable machine row at the gym, this is rowing for your actual life. Pull hard enough and you live. Slack off and you're tomorrow's buffet.

**The Exercise: Barbell/Dumbbell Row**

- Stand with feet shoulder-width apart, hinge at the hips, and let the weight hang at arm's length.

- Pull the weight toward your torso, elbows tight, squeezing your back like you're slamming a bunker door.

- Lower slowly, because control beats chaos, even during the apocalypse.

**Prescription:**

- 4–5 sets of 8–10 reps.

- Rest 90 seconds between sets (or however long it takes to check for bite marks).

- Bonus: Use odd objects (sandbags, crates, or backpacks) for "authentic survival vibes."

**Form Tips:**

- Keep your back flat; hunching here is a one-way ticket to your "undead chiropractor."

- Drive elbows straight back, not out, unless you're trying to clothesline invisible zombies.

- Brace your core like your future depends on it, because it does.

**Just A Tip:**
If the door doesn't budge, just yell, *"Functional fitness, my ass!"* and prepare to run.

## The Bridge Block Car Push

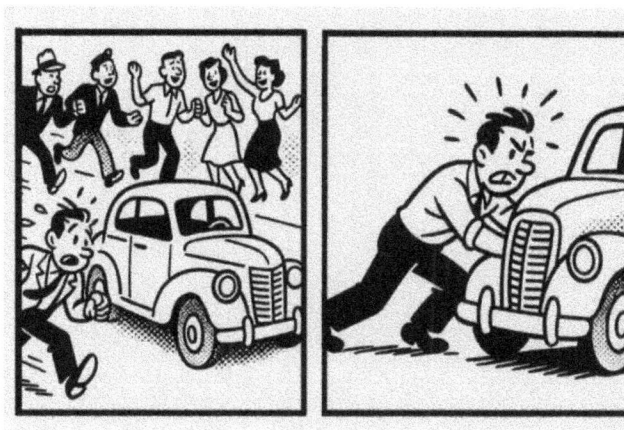

**Scenario:**

The apocalypse is here, and the only way out of town is across a narrow bridge. Problem is, there's a car jammed sideways, blocking the path like a giant middle finger to your survival.

Behind you: zombies. Below you: a frigid, rushing river that guarantees hypothermia faster than you can say "bad decision." Your options are simple: get bitten, freeze to death, or summon the leg power of a thousand squats and push this car out of the way. Choose wisely.

**The Exercise: Sled Push**

- Load a sled (or imagine the apocalypse-mobile blocking your bridge) with challenging weight.

- Lean into it, hands low, back flat, core braced.

- Drive forward with short, powerful steps, pushing like your life depends on it, because it does.

**Prescription:**

- 4–6 pushes of 20–40 yards.

- Rest 90–120 seconds between sets (time to "scan for zombies").

- Bonus: Try adding uneven weight to mimic the chaos of pushing a busted-up car at a bad angle.

**Form Tips:**

- Stay low, upright posture is for people who don't want to live.

- Drive with your legs, not your arms; arms steer, legs survive.

- Keep your breathing steady; panic burns fuel faster than cardio.

**Just A Tip:**

If you ever practice this in real life and someone asks why, just growl, *"Bridge clearance drill."* They will become confused and won't stick around for follow-up questions.

## The Last Door Sledge

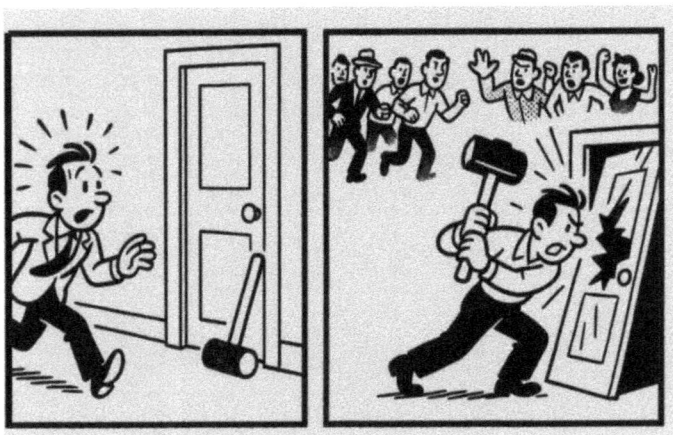

**Scenario:**
The horde is closing in. You've sprinted, dodged, and prayed, only to find yourself face-to-face with a locked, reinforced door. On the other side? Safety. On your side? A wall of undead ready to make you their midnight snack.

Your only option: grab the nearest sledgehammer and start swinging like your survival is sponsored by your local hardware store. Every slam buys you a second closer to escape and a second further from becoming zombie chow.

**The Exercise: Sledgehammer Slams**

- Grab a sledgehammer (or weighted substitute).

- Stand with feet shoulder-width apart, hammer overhead.

- Drive it down in a powerful arc, slamming into a tire, pad, or safe surface.

- Reset and repeat, imagining the sound of groaning zombies right behind you.

**Prescription:**

- 5–6 rounds of 15–20 slams.

- Rest 60–90 seconds between rounds (check your "perimeter" during breaks).

- Bonus: Alternate sides to balance the carnage, zombies won't care if you're lopsided, but we do.

**Form Tips:**

- Keep your core braced; sloppy swings end with you knocked out, not breaking free.

- Use hips and shoulders together for power, not just arms.

- Control the rebound, sledgehammers are loyal to no one. (Seriously, your shins will thank you.)

**Just A Tip:**
If someone asks why you're smashing a tire in the gym, just whisper, *"Zombies,"* and get back to work.

**The Wall Escape**

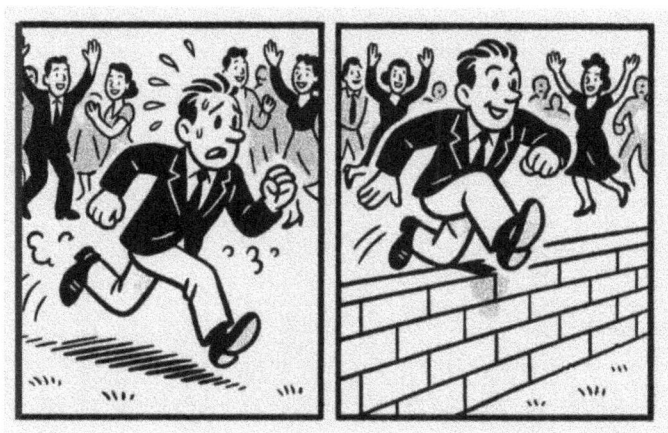

**Scenario:**

The street is swarming with zombies, and your only escape route is up and over a crumbling wall. There's no ladder, no stairs, and definitely no time to search the internet for the "best way to scale a wall."

You either pull yourself up and over like your life depends on it (because it does), or you become part of the horde's all-you-can-eat buffet. Welcome to the pull-up, your last shot at vertical freedom.

## The Exercise: Pull-Up / Rope Climb

- Grip a sturdy bar (or rope) with hands shoulder-width apart.

- Hang with arms straight, core tight, resisting the urge to kick like a fish out of water.

- Pull your chest toward the bar (or climb hand-over-hand), driving elbows down and back.

- Clear the bar/wall/imaginary salvation, then lower with control. Jumping down into a super hero landing is for the movies.

## Prescription:

- 4–6 sets of 3–8 reps (or climbs).

- Rest 2 minutes between sets. Real escapes won't allow it, but practice will.

- Bonus: Add a weighted vest or pack to simulate hauling your gear out with you.

**Form Tips:**

- Keep your chest tall and core braced; swinging wildly burns energy you don't have.

- Use your lats, not just your arms. This isn't "bicep bravado," it's survival engineering.

- If climbing rope, pinch with your legs; unless rope burn is the aesthetic you're going for.

**Just A Tip:**
If you can't get over the wall, just yell, *"Save yourselves!"* and accept your role as apocalypse distraction.

## The Endurance Escape

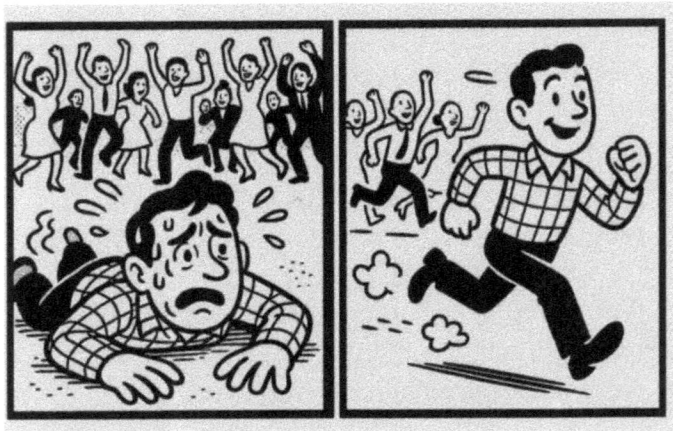

**Scenario:**
Here's the truth: you can swing a sledge, climb a wall, or push a car all you want, but if your heart gives out after 90 seconds, you're just another NPC for the horde. When the undead are everywhere, you don't need sprint speed, you need *endurance*: the ability to run far enough, long enough, and steady enough to reach safety without collapsing faster than your willpower around Nana's desserts. Zone 2 cardio is how you train to show up fresh, not fried, when the next fight for survival begins.

**The Exercise: Zone 2 Run**

- Find a steady pace you could hold while still talking (barely). Think "nervous small talk," not "last words."

- Keep your heart rate around 60–70% of your max.
    - (220-Your Age)*.6
    - Example: 220-40 = 180*.6 = 108 HR

- Run for distance or time, building gradually like your life depends on it (because it does).

**Prescription:**

- 2–3 sessions per week.

- Start with 20–30 minutes, progress toward 45–60.

- Bonus: Practice with a weighted vest or pack to mimic hauling supplies during an escape.

**Form Tips:**

- Run tall, hunching makes you look like you're already half-zombie.

- Keep your stride smooth; stomping burns energy and sounds like a dinner bell.

- Breathe steady through your nose when possible, panic breathing is cardio treason.

**Just A Tip:**
If anyone asks why you're jogging slow, just grin and laugh menacingly. They'll speed up. You'll outlast them.

## The Apocalypse Comfort Haul

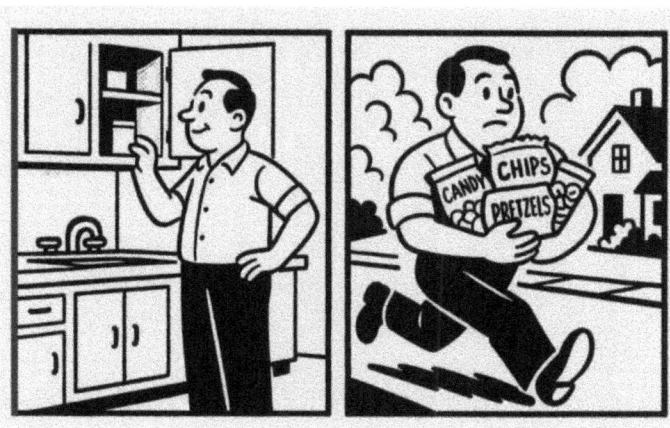

**Scenario:**
The world's ending, supplies are scarce, and every survival guide says the same thing: pack light, travel fast. But then you see it… your prized stand mixer. Or maybe it's the family-sized jar of your favorite chocolate spread. Or that giant box of snacks you swore you'd "ration." Rationally, you should leave it behind. Emotionally? You'd sooner fight the undead barehanded. So you hoist it to your chest in a weighted front carry, because sure, water and ammo matter, but so do brownies, peanut butter, and avoiding world ending hanger.

**The Exercise: Front Carry**

- Pick up a heavy, awkward object (sandbag, box of snacks, stand mixer, or yes, your apocalypse comfort item).

- Hug it tight to your chest like the last shred of civilization.

- Walk forward with small, steady steps, don't rush, wobble, or drop your lifeline.

- Keep your core braced, because nothing makes the apocalypse worse than low back pain and dropped snacks.

**Prescription:**

- 4–5 carries of 30–50 yards.

- Rest 90 seconds between carries or enough time to wipe that delicious cheesy orange dust off your hands.

- Bonus: Train with awkward, bulky objects (kitchen appliances, boxes, coolers) for "apocalypse mode".

**Form Tips:**

- Chest tall, if you hunch, you look like a sad raccoon protecting trash.

- Weight close, distance makes heavy feel heavier (and less heroic).

- Steady steps > stumbling sprint; apocalypse shame is eternal.

**Just A Tip:**

If anyone questions your choice of survival item, just look them dead in the eye and say, *"Nobody rebuilds society without snacks."*

# SECTION 7

## NEFARIOUS ACTIVITIES

# SECTION 7: NEFARIOUS ACTIVITIES

Not every workout is about health, longevity, or "functional fitness." Sometimes it's about poor decisions, questionable friends, and the kind of scenarios you'll never admit to in public.

This section is for those moments when the cops are chasing you, the body won't drag itself, and your buddy needs to be smuggled out of the bar before he starts another fight with the jukebox.

Here, training gets... suspicious. Vaulting fences when running isn't enough. Dragging heavy loads with a little too much practice. Balancing like a cat burglar so the floorboards don't rat you out. Hauling your friend like a sack of potatoes before the bouncers notice. And squeezing yourself through vents like an off-brand action hero who definitely skipped stunt training.

Will you ever need these skills? Hopefully not. Should you train them anyway? Absolutely. Because if life ever does drop you into a movie-level mess, at least you'll have the strength, balance, and questionable judgment to survive it.

Welcome to Nefarious Activities, don't ask, don't tell, just train.

## The Fence Flight

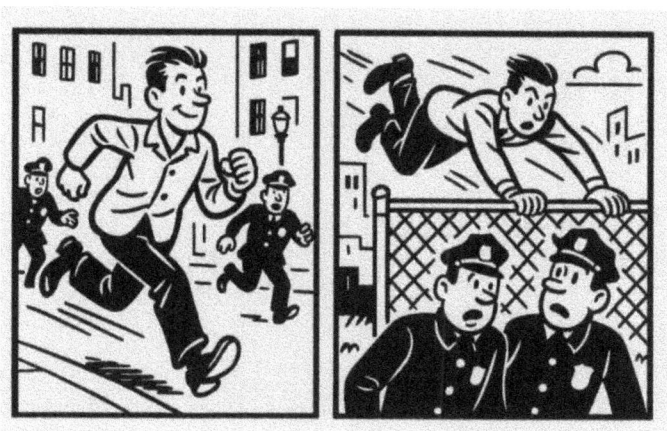

**Scenario:**
It all started as a harmless idea. Maybe it was graffiti, maybe it was "borrowing" a shopping cart for joyriding, maybe it was just running your mouth a little too loud at the wrong time. Now the cops are behind you, sirens wailing, and your brilliant plan has led you straight to a tall chain-link fence. Turning back isn't an option. Talking your way out isn't happening. The only choice is to vault this thing like your freedom depends on it, because, well, it does.

**The Exercise: Monkey Vault**

- Approach a sturdy box, platform, or rail (your "training fence").

- Place both hands firmly on the top edge.

- Jump explosively, driving your knees up as your feet leave the ground.

- Swing your legs to one side of your hands, clearing the obstacle in one smooth motion.

- Land softly on the other side and keep moving. Hesitation is how you end up explaining yourself to a judge.

**Prescription:**

- 4–6 sets of 5–8 vaults.

- Rest 90 seconds between sets. Recovery is a luxury you won't get mid-chase.

- Bonus: Practice with different heights, because fences in the wild come in all shapes and sizes.

**Form Tips:**

- Commit fully; half-hearted vaults end with you tangled in chain-link like a discount lawn ornament.

- Keep your weight over your hands for balance and speed.

- Bend your knees on landing, nothing kills momentum like faceplanting into freedom.

**Just A Tip:**
If you don't clear it on the first try, just yell *"Parkour!"* and hope the cops are too busy laughing to catch you.

## The Body Drag

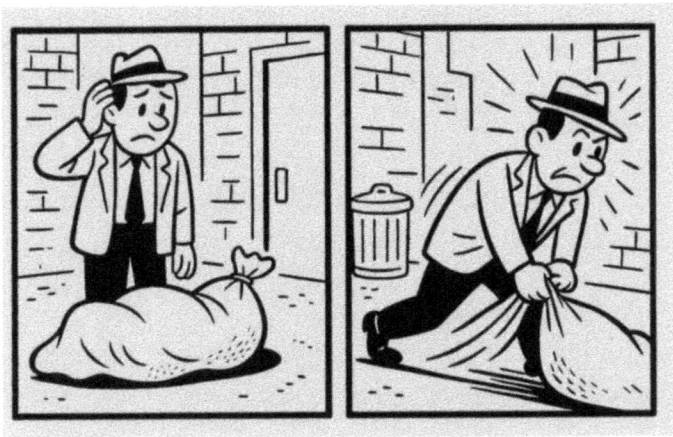

**Scenario:**
Look, we're not here to ask questions. Mistakes were made, and now you find yourself in the kind of situation where you've got to move something... quickly.

Discretion is key, noise is your enemy, and this load isn't walking itself out of here. Enter the sled drag, the perfect training for when you've got to haul something heavy, awkward, and potentially incriminating without blowing out your back.

## The Exercise: Sled Drag

- Attach straps or ropes to a weighted sled (or anything that slides).

- Face away from the sled, grab the handles, and start walking forward.

- Keep your steps smooth and steady, pulling with your legs and not your spine.

- Think "relaxed stroll," not "panicked sprint."

## Prescription:

- 4–6 sets of 30–50 yards.

- Rest 90 seconds between drags, or however long it takes to check if anyone's watching.

- Bonus: Try backward sled drags to balance out the legs. It's suspicious either way.

**Form Tips:**

- Keep your chest tall, you don't want to have bad form if you are caught in the act.

- Drive with your legs; yanking with your arms will leave you smoked in seconds.

- Steady pace > frantic jerks. Smooth criminals last longer.

**Just A Tip:**

If anyone asks why you're practicing this in public, just smile and say, *"Practicing for tonight."* Then wink. That'll clear the room fast.

## The Cat Burglar

**Scenario:**
You've made it inside. The dog is asleep, the floorboards are old, and the difference between success and disaster is one creak away. Every step has to be smooth, silent, and balanced, like a cat burglar gliding through the night. One wobble and the lights are on, alarms are blaring, and your career in questionably legal activities is over before it starts. Enter the single-leg Romanian deadlift: the perfect move for training balance, control, and tiptoeing over hardwood floors without sounding like a marching band.

**The Exercise: Single-Leg Romanian Deadlift**

- Stand tall with a weight (dumbbell, kettlebell, or "borrowed" vase) in one hand.

- Shift your weight to the opposite leg.

- Hinge forward at the hips, extending your free leg straight behind you like you're sneaking across a booby-trapped hallway.

- Lower the weight toward the floor with control, then return to standing without tipping over.

**Prescription:**

- 3–4 sets of 8–10 reps per leg.

- Rest 60–90 seconds between sets.

- Bonus: Train barefoot on creaky floors. Every professional practices before the big game.

**Form Tips:**

- Keep your back flat. Hunching makes you look more like a scared kitty instead of a smooth cat.

- Control the descent; jerky movements equal noisy floorboards.

- Keep your eyes fixed forward for balance or on the sleeping dog.

**Just A Tip:**
If you wobble mid-rep, don't worry you're just buffering. Do you think Ocean's 11 didn't stumble on the way to success?

## The Buddy Haul

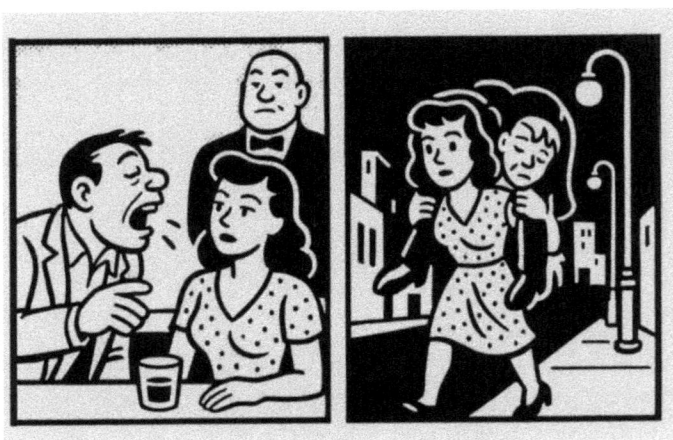

**Scenario:**
Your buddy said they'd "take it easy tonight." Several shots, 4 margaritas, and one too many bad one-liners later, they're drooling on their sleeve trying to tell you how they "totally have a shot with the bartender" and the bouncers are eyeballing your table like vultures circling a fresh carcass. You've got one shot to save your buddy's dignity and avoid the escorted walk of shame: hoist them over your shoulder and march them out like a one-man rescue squad. It's time for the fireman's carry, equal parts hero move and damage control.

## The Exercise: Fireman's Carry

- Start beside your buddy (or a weighted dummy).

- Squat down, hook one of their arms over your shoulder, and grab their opposite leg.

- Explosively stand, hoisting them across your shoulders like an awkward human backpack.

- Keep your core braced and walk steadily, bonus points if you don't drop them when they start singing.

## Prescription:

- 3–4 carries of 20–30 yards.

- Rest 2–3 minutes between sets (hydration breaks are optional, dropping your friend is not).

- Bonus: Practice with awkward weights, because no two drunk friends weigh the same.

**Form Tips:**

- Lift with your legs, not your back, otherwise you'll need your own rescue.

- Keep steps short and steady. When rescuing someone, we must adhere to the first rule.

- Balance matters; shift them mid-carry if they feel like a sack of potatoes.

**Just A Tip:**
If anyone asks why you're carrying your friend like a duffel bag, just say, *"Designated lifter."*

## The Vent Escape

**Scenario:**
The heist went sideways. Alarms are blaring, footsteps echo in the hall, and the only way out is through a ventilation shaft that looks like it was designed for raccoons, not humans. You jump, grab the edge, and now it's all on your abs to pull those legs up and squeeze into the duct before security kicks in the door. You're officially living the budget action movie life.

*Yippee Ki-Yay, m\*fer.*

**The Exercise: Hanging Leg Raise**

- Hang from a pull-up bar (or anything sturdy enough to hold your questionable decisions).

- Keep your arms straight, shoulders engaged, and core tight.

- Slowly lift your legs until they're parallel to the ground, like you're sneaking into a vent.

- Lower them back down under control, no wild swinging, this isn't CrossFit.

**Prescription:**

- 3–4 sets of 8–12 reps.

- Rest 60–90 seconds between sets (or however long it takes the imaginary guards to pass).

- Bonus: Add ankle weights or hold a medicine ball between your feet for "extra realism."

**Form Tips:**

- Don't yank yourself around; smooth, controlled lifts keep it stealthy.

- Engage your core, not just your hip flexors.

- Keep your grip strong, falling out of the "vent" ruins the escape.

**Just A Tip:**

If someone asks why you're hanging upside down at the gym, just mutter, *"Practicing my escape route."* In their confusion, you can make your escape.

# WHY FITNESS SHOULD BE FUN

If you've made it this far, congratulations, you now know how to scramble like a mountain goat, out-sprint angry geese, save your drunk friends, dispose of your enemies, and haul your snacks through the apocalypse. But here's the real takeaway: fitness doesn't have to be grim, joyless, or locked behind a wall of six-pack selfies and performance charts. Fitness can (and should) be playful.

When you let yourself laugh at the absurdity of training for geese, zombies, or shopping carts with four-wheel steering, you unlock something important: you stop seeing exercise as punishment, and start seeing it as practice for life's chaos. And life, as we both know, is nothing but chaos.

And let's not forget: laughing burns calories too. Sure, not as many as a sled push or a hill sprint, but combine a few sets of belly laughs with some burpees and you're practically a metabolic machine. If you're sweating and smiling, you're doing it right.

So here's the encouragement: keep moving. Not because the gym told you to, not because an influencer guilted you into it, but because life is full of absurd little challenges: chasing kids, carrying awkward loads, running late, climbing stairs, dodging elbows on dance floors... and the fitter you are, the more fun you'll have handling them. Strength and health are the ticket to living bigger, sillier, wilder lives.

And just in case you still want more – more challenge, more chaos, more story – we've saved one last gift for you. A bonus section of full-blown, story-based workouts where you'll step into the adventure itself: a strength quest, a power challenge, a balance trial, and an endurance circuit — all built to immerse you in the fun while still delivering serious fitness.

Because at the end of the day, fitness isn't just about reps and sets. It's about being ready for whatever life throws at you... angry goose, bar fight, or a tiny plastic brick minefield.

Now... get ready for the bonus round!

# BONUS WORKOUTS

## FOUR STORIES TO RULE THEM ALL

## Bonus Workout 1: Escape the Wreckage (Strength)

**Scenario:**
Your plane didn't exactly "land." It crash-introduced itself to the wilderness, leaving you surrounded by twisted metal, fallen beams, and supplies scattered everywhere. Survivors are looking at you like *you* have a plan. This is not the moment for curls or ab selfies. This is the moment for raw, brute strength — the kind that lifts, carries, and survives. Welcome to *Escape the Wreckage.*

**The Workout: Big Compound Survival Lifts**

**1. Deadlifts – Lift the Fallen Beam**

- Stand over a loaded barbell (or heavy object).

- Hinge at the hips, grip the bar, and drive through your heels to stand tall.

- Imagine you're pulling a beam off the wreckage, because you are.
  **Sets/Reps:** 4×6–8 heavy, controlled reps.

## 2. Overhead Press – Signal with a Flare / Lift Gear Overhead

- Rack the weight at your shoulders.

- Press straight overhead, arms locked out, core braced.

- Visualize holding a flare high enough for rescue… or just getting supplies into overhead storage.
  **Sets/Reps:** 4×8–10.

## 3. Farmer's Carries – Hauling Water Across Camp

- Grab heavy dumbbells, kettlebells, or jugs (bonus points if they slosh).

- Walk steadily, core braced, shoulders tall, like you're hauling precious water across camp.
  **Sets/Reps:** 4 carries of 40–50 yards.

### 4. Weighted Squats – Building the Base

- Load a barbell on your back (or hug a heavy object).

- Squat deep, drive back up strong.

- Think of it as training your legs to handle the constant load of survival life.
  **Sets/Reps:** 4×8–10.

**Benefit:**
This workout builds the kind of full-body strength that actually matters: picking up heavy things, pressing them overhead, carrying awkward loads, and squatting under pressure. Not only will you look stronger — you'll *be* stronger, the kind of person who doesn't crumble under debris, groceries, or apocalypse baggage.

**Just A Tip:**
If anyone asks what you're training for, just stare off dramatically and say, *"The crash. Always the crash."*

## Bonus Workout 2: The Great Getaway (Power)

**Scenario:**
The chase is on. Maybe it's cops, maybe it's zombies, maybe it's a flock of unreasonably angry geese. Doesn't matter. You don't need endurance, you need bursts of pure, explosive power. Every fence you clear, every escape you make, every slam you throw is one step closer to freedom. This isn't jogging in the park. This is survival in motion. Welcome to *The Great Getaway*.

**The Workout: Explosiveness Under Pressure**

**1. Box Jumps – Clearing Fences**

- Stand in front of a sturdy box or platform.

- Drop into a quarter squat, swing arms back, and explode up, landing soft and balanced.

- Picture the chain-link fence between you and your pursuers.
  **Sets/Reps:** 5×5 jumps.

## 2. Kettlebell Swings – Hip-Powered Escape

- Stand with feet shoulder-width, kettlebell in front.

- Hike it back, then drive through your hips to swing the bell to just above your navel.

- Think of it as building the hip power that launches you into every sprint, vault, or chaotic getaway.
  **Sets/Reps:** 4×12–15.

## 3. Burpee Broad Jump - Down but Not Out

- Drop your chest to the floor like you're being cuffed.

- Explosively leap up and jump out of the way, like a gazelle evading the sweet embrace of death from a hungry lion.

- Now do it again and again. Try not to hate me for this one. **Sets/Reps:** 4×10–12 (5–6 each side).

## 4. Medicine Ball Slams – The Frustration Release

- Start with a medicine ball overhead.

- Slam it to the ground like you're crushing every obstacle in your way.

- Scoop it up and repeat, channeling all your panic and rage into the floor.
  **Sets/Reps:** 4×10–12.

**Benefit:**

This workout builds explosive speed you need to evade capture from anyone who may or may not be involved in your alleged activities. You'll be ready to leap, dodge, vault, and slam your way out of any pursuit, real or imagined.

**Just A Tip:**

It's prison rules for those Kettlebell Swings. Clench your glutes tight. Best to be prepared if you get caught… we recommend not getting caught.

## Bonus Workout 3: The Cat Burglar (Balance & Agility)

**Scenario:**
It's late at night. The building is quiet. You're dressed in black, sneaking past creaky floorboards, darting through invisible laser grids, and tiptoeing your way across rooftops that definitely weren't designed for this. One wrong move and you're either caught, alarmed, or falling through someone's ceiling mid-mission. To survive as a proper cat burglar, you'll need balance, agility, and the ability to move like a shadow.

**The Workout: Silent but Deadly (in a Good Way)**

**1. Single-Leg Romanian Deadlifts – Quiet Tiptoeing**

- Stand tall with a weight in one hand.

- Balance on the opposite leg, hinge at the hips, and lower the weight with control.

- Return to standing without wobbling, like you're sneaking across floorboards that squeak louder than your getaway van's suspension.
  **Sets/Reps:** 3–4×8–10 per leg.

## 2. Lateral Bounds – Dodging Invisible Lasers

- Balance on one leg, then explosively leap sideways to land on the other.

- Stick the landing softly, knees bent, like you just dodged a glowing tripwire.
  **Sets/Reps:** 4×10–12 (5–6 per side).

## 3. Plank Shoulder Taps – The Stealth Crawl

- Start in a high plank, hands under shoulders.

- Tap one shoulder with the opposite hand, keeping hips as steady as possible.

- Imagine crawling silently under a laser grid while holding your breath.
  **Sets/Reps:** 3–4×12–16 taps.

## 4. Agility Ladder Drills – Darting Rooftops

- Set up an agility ladder (or mark spaces on the ground).

- Perform quick, precise footwork patterns: in-and-outs, lateral shuffles, or high knees.

- Picture yourself sprinting across a rooftop, rooftop cat mode fully engaged.
  **Sets/Reps:** 4–5 drills, 20–30 seconds each.

**Benefit**:
This workout builds balance, coordination, and core stability. Translation: fewer wobbles, smoother movements, and the kind of sneaky control that lets you get through life's "laser grids" (or just your kid's toy minefield) without incident.

**Just A Tip:**
If anyone asks why you're doing agility drills at night, just whisper, *"Can't talk... mission in progress."*

## Bonus Workout 4: The Gauntlet (Endurance Circuit)

**Scenario:**
This is it. The ultimate test. You've been chased, cornered, and dropped into the mother of all obstacle courses. Alarms are blaring, shadows are closing in, and your only way out is to keep moving — fast, efficient, and relentless. No breaks, no excuses. Every obstacle is waiting for you: walls to climb, floors to crawl, loads to carry, and sprints to escape. Survive *The Gauntlet* and you're not just fit — you're legend.

**The Workout: Circuit of Chaos**

Perform each exercise back-to-back with minimal rest. Complete 3–5 full rounds.

**1. Burpees – Hit the Deck, Pop Back Up**

- Drop, hit the floor, pop back up, and leap into the air.
- Think: dodging a sudden attack or diving under lasers. **Reps:** 12–15.

## 2. Pull-Ups / Inverted Rows – Wall Escape

- Grip a bar, pull yourself up (or under) with control.

- Picture scaling that wall before the horde catches up. **Reps:** 8–10.

## 3. Sandbag or Dumbbell Front Carry – Hauling the Supplies

- Hug a heavy weight to your chest and walk steady.

- This is your lifeline; water, food, or maybe just snacks. **Distance:** 40 yards (or 30–40 seconds).

## 4. Mountain Climbers – Low Profile Endurance

- High plank, knees driving toward your chest, fast and furious.

- You're crawling under alarms and through tight vents. **Reps:** 40 total (20 per side).

## 5. Sprint – Final Escape

- Give it everything. Short, sharp burst of speed.

- Imagine the exit is right there, don't slow down.
  **Distance/Time:** 50–100 yards (or 20–30 seconds).

**Benefit:**
This circuit builds the ultimate survival package: endurance, speed, strength under fatigue, and the grit to keep moving no matter how absurd the situation. It's the closest thing to real-life chaos training, minus the actual alarms, lasers, and security guards.

**Just A Tip:**
If you collapse mid-circuit, just wheeze out, *"Tell my story,"* and know you've earned it.

## THOUGHTS BEFORE YOU GO

So here we are, the end of the book. By now you've trained for geese, zombies, bouncers, poorly designed shopping carts, toddlers, sharks, and the occasional questionable life decision.

You've deadlifted wreckage, vaulted fences, carried buddies, hauled snacks, and maybe even whispered "mission in progress" during plank shoulder taps. In short: you're no longer just exercising. You're preparing for life's absurdities.

Here's something to really take home, fitness isn't about perfection. It's not about looking like an influencer or grinding yourself into dust. It's about having fun, laughing at the chaos, and showing up consistently enough that when life inevitably throws something ridiculous your way, you're ready.

Because it *will*. The stroller will roll toward traffic. The dance floor will turn hostile. The dog will put the toy in the hardest to reach spot under the couch. And yes, one day you might even have to push a car to help a stranger (or yourself) or vault a fence you had no business climbing.

If you keep moving, keep laughing, and keep showing up, you won't just be fit, you'll be confident and capable. Strong enough for the heavy stuff, agile enough for the weird stuff, and resilient enough for all the stuff in between.

So take these workouts, enjoy them, and don't take yourself too seriously. Because at the end of the day, fitness should make you smile just as much as it makes you sweat.

Be playful. Be consistent. Be ready.

# Appendix A: Warm-Up, Cool-Down & Scaling

Before you start vaulting fences, dragging sleds, or smuggling friends out of bars, let's talk about the unglamorous but necessary stuff: warming up, cooling down, and scaling. Think of this as the duct tape of fitness– it's not flashy, but it keeps everything from falling apart.

## Warm-Up (5–8 Minutes)

Your body isn't a light switch. Don't just walk in cold and jump into burpees, unless your goal is to experience regret at high speed.

### Step 1: Wake Up the System (2–3 minutes)

- Brisk walk, easy jog, or bike at "I can still text while doing this" pace.

### Step 2: Dynamic Prep (2 rounds)

- 10 Bodyweight Squats (hips and knees inline)
- 10 Arm Circles per side (wake up the shoulders)
- 10 Hip Hinges (practice not looking like a folding chair)
- 20-Second Plank (abs and brain engaged)

## Cool-Down (3–5 Minutes)

Think of this as closing out the mission report. Bring the heart rate down and convince your muscles you don't hate them.

### Step 1: Slow It Down (2 minutes)

- Easy walk or slow pedal, deep breaths in and out.

### Step 2: Stretch the Trouble Spots (30–60 seconds each)

- Calves (because stairs are everywhere)
- Hips (squats, lunges, life in general)
- Lats/Shoulders (all the carrying, all the time)

## Scaling Rules (a.k.a. Don't Die Doing This)

### Rule 1: Range Beats Load

- Full, clean movement > stacking weight like you're auditioning for a strongman show.

### Rule 2: The Talk Test

- If you can't say a sentence without gasping, you're sprinting. Save that for angry goose day.

### Rule 3: Swap Smart, Not Lazy

- Pull-Ups → Ring Rows or Band-Assisted Pull-Ups

- Box Jumps → Step-Ups

- Burpees → Down-Up (no push-up/jump)

- Running → Bike/Row at same time effort

**Rule 4: Respect the Twinge**

- Sharp pain ≠ badass. It ≠ progress. It ≠ "just push through." Stop, scale, and live to fight another goose.

**Just A Tip:**

If anyone makes fun of you for scaling, ignore them. They don't know what they are talking about, or they are just an ass. *You do you, Boo Boo.*

# Appendix B: The 4-Week On-Ramp

Starting a new routine is like sneaking into a laser-grid vault, if you rush it, you're toast. This 4-week plan eases you in, helps you learn the moves, and builds enough strength, endurance, and coordination to handle whatever absurdity life throws at you.

**Schedule:**

2–3 sessions per week. Non-consecutive days. Think "Monday-Wednesday-Friday," not "three nights in a row and then collapse."

**Week 1: Learn the Moves**

- **Day 1:**
    - Suitcase Carry (3×30 yards/side)
    - Bodyweight Squats (3×10)
    - Plank Hold (3×20 sec)
- **Day 2:**
    - Step-Ups (3×8/leg)
    - Single-Leg RDL (light, 3×8/leg)
    - Calf Raises (3×12)

**Mission:** Get comfortable, not cocky. This is reconnaissance.

**Week 2: Add Some Spice**

- **Day 1:**
    - Burpees (scaled if needed, 3×6–8)
    - Forward Lunges (3×8/leg)
    - Side Plank (3×20 sec/side)
- **Day 2:**
    - Farmer's Hold (3×30 sec)
    - Bear Crawl (3×20 yards)
    - Inverted Rows or Ring Rows (3×8–10)

**Mission:** Test your balance and grit. Nothing too heavy…yet.

**Week 3: Build the Base**

- **Day 1:**
    - Deadlift (light barbell, kettlebell, or sandbag, 4×6)
    - Suitcase Carry (4×30 yards/side)
- **Day 2:**
    - Pull-Ups (or band/ring rows, 3×6–8)
    - Agility Shuffle (3×20 sec)
    - Push-Ups (3×8–12)

**Mission:** Handle more load without crumbling. Think "I'm new, but I'm enthusiastic!"

## Week 4: Test the System

- **Day 1:**
    - Overhead Press (4×8)
    - Turkish Get-Up (light, 3×3/side)
    - Calf Raises (4×12)
- **Day 2:** Mini-Circuit (5 rounds, rest as needed):
    - 5 Burpees
    - 20-Second Farmer's Carry
    - 20-Second Sprint

**Mission:** Put it all together. The goal isn't to collapse, it's to control the chaos.

## Progression Rule of Thumb:

- Add **1–2 reps** or **a little weight** each week, not both.

- If you're scaling, that's not weakness — it's strategy. Every cat burglar starts with baby steps.

**Just A Tip:**

If you feel sore after week one, congratulations, you're alive. If you're not sore after week four, congratulations, you're dangerous.

# Appendix C: Minimal Equipment Kit

Here's the truth: you don't need a $5,000 home gym to train for angry geese, toddlers, foot destroying toy mines, or bar buddy extractions. You just need a few tools that can double as apocalypse survival gear. Keep it simple, keep it portable, and you'll always be ready.

## The Core Kit (covers 90% of this book)

- **Kettlebell or Dumbbells (1–2 sizes):** Your all-in-one tool. Swings, carries, presses, deadlifts, basically your survival cannon ball with a handle.
- **Resistance Bands + Door Anchor:** Cheap, packable, and perfect for rows, pulls, or strapping yourself to things you shouldn't.
- **Pull-Up Bar:** Doorway or mounted. Essential for wall escapes, vents, and shark-avoidance practice.
- **Sturdy Box/Step:** Step-ups, jumps, vault practice. Does not have to be fancy. Bonus points if it doesn't wobble.
- **Sandbag or Duffel Bag:** Load it with rice, mulch, or your embarrassingly large collection of Beanie Babies. Hug, carry, squat, and drag the king of awkward weights.

## The Nice-to-Have Add-Ons

- **Jump Rope:** Cheap cardio, portable, and great for pretending you're preparing to fight Ivan Drago.
- **Agility Ladder (or sidewalk chalk):** Footwork drills. Makes you look like you're planning a heist….or playing hopscotch.
- **Medicine Ball:** For slams, throws, and working out stress before it builds into felony charges.
- **Weighted Vest or Backpack:** Fill with books, bricks, or water jugs. Perfect for rucking, carries, and feeling unstoppable.

## DIY / Household Substitutes

- **Grocery Bags:** Suitcase carry. Bonus: you're already training for "one trip or die trying."
- **Chairs:** Dips, step-ups, or barricading the hallway when the kids go feral.
- **Buckets of Water / Cat Litter:** Instant farmer's carry gear. Just don't spill them.
- **Couch Cushions:** Agility drills, fall training, nap recovery.

**Golden Rule:**

It doesn't matter if it's store bought shiny or homemade; if it's heavy, awkward, or makes you sweat, it works.

**Just A Tip:**
If anyone side-eyes your "homemade sandbag," just mutter, *"Prototype. Not for civilians."* They will be confused, possibly intrigued, and now you have a business to make money to buy new gear.

# Appendix D: Glossary of Terms

**Agility** – The ability to move fast, change direction, and not trip over your own feet. Think dodging invisible lasers or your crazy aunt on the dance floor.

**Brace** – Tighten your core like someone's about to poke you in the ribs. Protects your spine and makes you look serious.

**Carry** – Walking with weight. Could be groceries, car seats, or a drunk friend. Builds grip, core, and pride.

**Compound Lift** – Big, multi-joint movement (deadlift, squat, press). The opposite of "tiny curls in the mirror."

**Core Stability** – Keeping your midsection steady so you don't flop like a loose spring during planks, carries, or life.

**DOMS** – Delayed Onset Muscle Soreness. Translation: the pain that shows up the day *after* you decide to work out. Not always necessary for progress, but it is an indicator you are working hard.

**Endurance** – The ability to keep going. Think running from zombies… for more than 30 seconds.

**Explosive Power** – Fast, all-out strength. The "jump the fence now or else" kind.

**Functional Fitness** – Training that actually helps you in life (lifting logs, hauling kids, pushing cars), not just looking cool on Instagram.

**Hinge** – Moving at the hips while keeping your back flat. Deadlift pattern. Practice this so you stop hurting yourself picking up socks.

**Isometric** – An exercise where you hold still under tension (plank, wall sit). Basically, suffering without moving.

**Mobility** – How easily your joints move. Important for hikers, burglars, and anyone who wants to squat without sounding like bubble wrap.

**NPC** – Short for Non-Playable character. IE, the extras that get offed easily in any TV show or movie. Popularized from video game culture.

**Plyometric** – Fancy word for jump training. Anything where you explode off the ground and hope to land on your feet.

**RPE (Rate of Perceived Exertion)** – Scale of 1–10 for effort. 1 = "walking to the fridge." 10 = "Angry goose is winning."

**Scaling** – Adjusting an exercise so you can actually do it without dying. Step-ups instead of box jumps, banded pull-ups instead of flailing.

**Unilateral** – One side at a time. Single-leg, single-arm. Builds balance and exposes which side is secretly useless.

**Zone 2** – Easy-steady cardio where you can hold a conversation. Train here to last longer than your neighbor when the geese attack.

**Just One Last Tip:**
If you forget any of these, don't panic. Just do the thing, sweat a little, and make up new terms. That's how half the fitness industry works anyway.

## SCAN ME FOR BONUSES

 Congrats, you survived *Fitness for the Absurd*. Now claim your reward before a goose steals it. Go to

**https://kokorohealthandfitness.com/fitness-for-the-absurd-bonuses** for the free bonus program Absurdly Fit: a 90-Day Mission to Strength, Sanity, and Survival and the official Absurd Snack Contingency Plan.

---

You've finished the book, survived the workouts, and possibly avoided minor injuries. Now, do one last rep, the review rep.

Go to Amazon, tap those stars, and tell the world how *Fitness for the Absurd* changed your life (or at least made you snort coffee out your nose).

Your review keeps this ridiculous movement alive. Literally.

# ABOUT THE AUTHOR

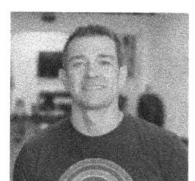 Josiah Miller (Joe) is a certified personal trainer, gym owner, and U.S. Navy veteran with nearly two decades of experience in fitness and wellness.

His unique approach combines real-world experience from military service and some admittedly absurd civilian adventures, that he may or may not have taken part in, with practical, no-nonsense training methods that actually work.

Over the years, Joe has seen how complicated and extreme the fitness world has become. Between influencer diets, 30-day miracles, and the "no excuses" mentality, people have forgotten that exercise is supposed to make life easier — not more stressful. Frustrated by the noise, he built his philosophy around one simple truth: fitness should prepare you for real life, and real life is rarely black and white.

This book exists because a client asked a simple question during a workout: "Do you write these scenarios down or just make them up on the fly?" The answer was "on the fly," followed by a joke about writing a book. A couple days later the idea hit him harder than taco night before leg day—he actually should write this damn book.

Joe owns and operates Kokoro Health and Fitness in Atlantic Beach, FL, where he continues to help people get fit while keeping them entertained.

www.ingramcontent.com/pod-product-compliance
Lightning Source LLC
Chambersburg PA
CBHW052129030426
42337CB00028B/5086